SIMPLE PRINCIPLES™
TO FEEL BETTER
& LIVE LONGER

Alex A. Lluch
Author of Over 3 Million Books Sold!

Dr. Helen Eckmann
Doctor of Education and Leadership Science

WS Publishing Group
San Diego, California

SIMPLE PRINCIPLES™
TO FEEL BETTER & LIVE LONGER

By Alex A. Lluch and Dr. Helen Eckmann

Published by WS Publishing Group
San Diego, California 92119
Copyright © 2008 by WS Publishing Group

Designed by WS Publishing Group:
David Defenbaugh

For Inquiries:
Logon to www.WSPublishingGroup.com
E-mail info@WSPublishingGroup.com

ISBN 13: 978-1-934386-08-8

Printed in China

TABLE OF CONTENTS

INTRODUCTION

People have sought ways to lengthen their lives for thousands of years. Throughout history, men have consulted oracles, gods, apothecaries, and even looked to the stars to find the magical secret that would bless them with a longer life. *Simple Principles™ to Feel Better & Live Longer* provides you with the many secrets to longer life that have eluded so many for so long.

Many people believe their life span is limited by the genetics they have inherited — that little can change the amount of time they will live or improve the quality of those days. Nothing could be further from the truth! Every single person can make changes to their lifestyle that will result in feeling their best every single day. Such changes will also result in added days, months, years, and even decades to their life!

The best thing about learning how to feel better is that once you do, you never want to go back. Once you get a taste of what it feels like to live a healthier, happier, and pain-free life, you become unable to go back to your old habits that kept you unhappy and unhealthy. To attain this blissful state, we need only to tap into the various sources within us to raise our level of consciousness regarding the steps that can be taken to result in longer life. At the same time, we must quiet the desires within us that promise to shorten our life span, such as eating poorly, smoking, and exposing ourselves to toxins. In other words, the key to living a better, longer life is to replace our tendency to do our bodies harm with a desire to feel better and live longer. *Simple Principles™ to Feel Better & Live Longer* emphasizes how to achieve this balance.

What is this book about?

In short, this is a book about feeling better each day and living a longer, fuller life. This is a book about increasing your quality of life and extending the number of days you live by making changes to your mind, body, and lifestyle. It is about learning new skills, including eating right, exercising properly, getting enough sleep, avoiding toxins and risky behaviors, and keeping yourself hydrated and limber. This book also offers information on how being a more sensual, spiritual, and social person can help you feel better and live longer, and it includes the ways that you can prevent illness, cope with sadness, and look, feel, and think young in order to reach this goal. Finally, this book is about maximizing your health, self-esteem, mental faculties, and environment to result in a more fulfilling, more productive, and longer-living you. Use this book as a tool to help you lead a longer, happier, and healthier life.

It is important to remember that life is a series of ups and downs. It is impossible to feel great every day out of the year. However, there is much you can do to maximize your number of good days and also the number of days you live overall. Before you start, however, it is important to recognize the things about your that cannot be changed and factor them into your plan of action. For example, you cannot change the fact that you have a history of heart disease in your family, but you can change your diet and lifestyle to minimize your risk of having heart troubles. This book will help you evaluate where to concentrate your energy in your quest for a longer and more satisfying life.

This book emphasizes the role that positive thinking and healthy lifestyle play in your overall quality of life. Several principles included in this book guide you away from destructive, unhealthy, or unproductive behaviors. There are also principles to help you learn how to change your mind about your abilities and circumstances. Finally, there are principles that offer scientific proof about how to extend your life that are so compelling, you will immediately want to change the way you live!

Who should read this book?

This book is for people who want to:

- Eat healthy, life-extending foods
- Learn which products contain life-threatening toxins
- Avoid behaviors that will reduce life span
- Learn how developing a spiritual side can make you feel better and live longer
- Learn to avoid heart disease and cancer
- Learn the benefits of getting a good night's sleep

- Learn why drinking water is one of the most important things you can do for yourself
- Practice relaxation and stress-reduction techniques
- Learn tools for coping with sadness
- Experience the benefits of nurturing relationships
- Look, think, and feel young
- Stimulate the mind to prevent aging diseases
- Stave off diseases such as cancer, osteoporosis, heart disease, and diabetes
- Understand how a healthy sex life can extend your life
- Develop and maintain a positive outlook
- Learn habits to help you feel good in both mind and body

Lastly, this book is for people who want to be able to flip to a page in a book that applies to their situation and find a quick inspirational tip that will quickly put them on the road to feeling better and living longer.

Why should you read this book?

Well, there is a reason why you were drawn to the title. But the fact is that everyone should read this book. Even if you consider yourself to be a happy and healthy person, there is something in here for you. You should read this book because it combines a lot of wisdom into easy-to-read simple principles. If you want to change your life and become a much healthier person who has the chance to live well into old age, you should read this book.

Here are some questions to ask yourself:

- Are you tired of feeling tired?
- Do you want to exercise but can never find the time?
- Do you feel uncomfortable in your body?
- Do you worry your lifestyle is leading you to an early grave?
- Are you a soda and junk-food fiend?
- Is it impossible for you to relax?
- Have you lost someone you loved?
- Are you satisfied with your relationships?
- Does fear prevent you from trying new things?
- Do you worry you will someday develop cancer or heart disease?
- Are you worried you look older than you actually are?

- Do you feel like you don't have the energy for life?
- Is it difficult for you to be intimate with your partner?
- Do you have a problem finding enjoyment?
- Do you miss the zest you once had for life?

If any of these questions resonate with you, read on. These are just a few of the many topics covered in this book. The principles contained in this book are researched and supported with inspirational quotes and statistical information from credible sources. Its size makes it easy to keep with you for easy reference or for a quick pick-me-up in the middle of the day. You should read this book whenever you are ready to make changes and improve your overall outlook on life.

LIVING A LONG
AND HEALTHY LIFE

Everyone wants to lead a pain-free, longer life complete with loving relationships, satisfying work, and an overall sense of happiness. So why is it so hard for many of us? One major obstacle is the fact that many people believe it is impossible to feel better and live longer. They think genetics are the only thing that affects the amount of time they are able to live and that very little can improve the quality of those days. This is untrue, of course. All it takes to feel better and live longer is the willingness to make a few basic lifestyle changes and the commitment to rewiring your mind and body for pleasure and long life.

What are the challenges to living a long and healthy life?

In addition to believing such a change is impossible, people feel overwhelmed by how much information they would need to change their lives to feel better and live longer. In fact, when asked to explain the reasons why they have given up on pursuing such a life, people usually comment, "I don't know where to start."

Make no mistake, changing your life to have a better and longer existence is a serious undertaking. It requires educating yourself on dietary, exercise, and lifestyle choices that will protect you from harm, disease, and depression. And as our world is increasingly filled with pollution, toxins, and other harmful substances, this is a difficult task. But *Simple Principles™ to Feel Better & Live Longer* arms you with the tools you need to give yourself the healthy edge, and in a fraction of the time had you attempted this on your own. This book takes volumes of research, statistics, anecdotes, and quotable wisdom and distills it down to bite-sized pieces of information you can understand, remember, and read quickly and easily. Indeed, reading this book is the first, and possibly the most important, step you can take toward getting control of your life and increasing your health and happiness. It makes feeling better and living longer easy, enjoyable, and completely within your grasp.

Why should you seek a long and healthy life?

Most people can agree that living a long and healthy life is obviously preferable to living a short and miserable one. But let's explore what a day in a healthy, long life is really like. It is a day in which you wake up feeling refreshed from an excellent night's sleep. It is a day in which you eat healthy meals packed with cancer-fighting vitamins and minerals that prevent your arteries from clogging and your bones from decaying. It is a day in which you make time to exercise, knowing that exercise prevents disease, cancer, and helps you look and feel decades younger than you are. It is a day in which, because you meditate and are in touch with your spiritual side, you feel relaxed and immune to the stresses and pressures of the world. It is a day in which you are aware of what products to avoid because of the levels of dangerous toxins they contain. It is a day in which you solve an interesting puzzle, indulge in a hobby or craft, or make time for intimacy with your partner. It is a day in which you take measures to prevent yourself from suffering the pain of a debilitating disease such as cancer or stroke. It is a day in which you have plans with a close friend, because you understand that having a network of friends is so satisfying that it extends life by at least half a decade. Finally, it is a day in which you avoid risky behaviors out of respect for the body and mind you have worked so hard to cultivate. You go to sleep after this fantastic day feeling emotionally satisfied, well-nourished, physically pain-free, and excited to see what tomorrow holds.

That's not a bad day, is it?

What do you need to know to live a long and healthy life?

There is a lot you will need to know in order to start living a long and healthy life, and this book simplifies the enormous amount of information for you. It offers the following tools to help you feel better and live longer:

- A diet to maximize your life span
- Tips for avoiding dangerous toxins
- Reasons to stop practicing risky behaviors
- Exercises that teach self-esteem and happiness
- How to replace negative thoughts with positive thoughts

- Ways to de-stress your life
- How to keep your body's systems healthy
- How to minimize your risk of cancer, heart attacks, stroke, and other disease
- Ways to explore your faith
- The connection between your physical and emotional health
- The importance of giving time to the people you care about
- Tools for coping with sadness
- Ways to keep your mind sharp

This book also will teach you that:

- Controlling your stress directly affects your ability to live a long life
- Drinking water is possibly the best thing to do for your body
- It is critically important to get enough rest
- Your perspective is everything
- Learning to cope with sadness does not devalue your loss
- You can extend your life by changing your behaviors

- Looking, feeling, and thinking young is within your grasp, no matter your age
- Debilitating illness such as cancer and diabetes can be prevented

Use the simple principles in this book as you would tools in a toolbox. Refer to them often as you need them. Eventually the tips in this book will become second nature, and you will automatically be living a life in which you naturally feel better every day.

Maximizing the Benefits of This Book

Always keep this book handy. Put it in the glove compartment of your car. Stick it in the top drawer of your desk at work. Lay it on your nightstand before bed. This book is written to be read over and over again. The principles will take time to affect change, so the idea is to read and practice them often. Remember that your pursuit for a longer, happier, and healthier life is a long-term goal that will take time and effort. However, you will feel better almost immediately once you start reading this book.

EATING RIGHT

Eating a healthy, well-balanced diet has been consistently found to have enormous health advantages. Yet a healthy diet hinges on the concept of moderation; that is, striking the right balance when consuming any one food or drink. Too much or too little of any one substance can have very different, and even harmful, effects.

An excellent example of the way in which moderation is important is red wine. Red wine is an alcoholic beverage containing about 18.75 mL of alcohol per 5 oz. glass. Excess amounts of alcohol in any form have been linked to the development of certain cancers, including cancer of the digestive tract, esophagus, mouth, larynx, liver, stomach, pancreas, lungs, breast, and colon.

But in moderation, red wine has been proven to have astonishing health benefits. In 1991, French scientist Serge

Renaud discovered them when he stumbled upon the French Paradox. The French Paradox is the reality that despite the fact that the French eat large amounts of heart-clogging saturated fats, smoke profusely, and exercise very little, they have one of the lowest rates of coronary heart disease in the world.

Renaud studied 34,000 middle-aged men living in eastern France who ate a normal French diet heavy in meats, cheeses, and red wine. He found that 2 to 3 glasses of red wine a day reduced the men's death rates from all causes by up to 30 percent. The alcohol and antioxidants present in the wine protect the heart from disease and also work to fight other cancers. His results were published in the journal *Epidemiology*, and of them he said, "I've always suspected this. Wine protects not only against heart disease but also most cancers."

So, how is it possible that in some cases red wine causes cancer and in other cases protects against it? The answer is that a substance in moderation can have very different effects than when consumed in excess. Soy is another example of how important it is to eat certain foods in moderation. Soy

how important it is to eat certain foods in moderation. Soy contains omega-3 fatty acids, which prevent heart disease and stroke. Soy also contains phytochemicals that prevent certain types of cancer. But when soy is eaten in large amounts by women predisposed to breast cancer, it can actually encourage the development of that cancer.

The health benefits of certain foods will continue to be researched, but the most important lessons to learn is that everything you consume must be in moderation. And no matter what a new study finds, the best dietary recommendations are also the most consistent: that getting adequate sources of vitamins, minerals, and antioxidants through foods are the best way to stay healthy. The following simple principles will help you figure out changes to make to your diet to start eating right immediately.

Principle #1

Fighting cancer with food.

Many fruits and vegetables are rich in cancer-fighting compounds known as antioxidants and phytochemicals. These compounds work by combating elements known as free radicals, which have been linked to cancer. Foods with antioxidants include tomatoes, berries, grapes, and spinach. Another cancer-fighting food is broccoli, which contains phytochemicals that are believed to make cancer cells less toxic. Tea, especially green tea, also contains phytochemicals, and has been associated with a lower risk of stomach, esophageal, and liver cancers. Studies suggest that people who eat foods rich in antioxidants and phytochemicals can **reduce** their risk of developing cancer by up to 50 percent.

PRINCIPLE #2

Eat your way to a healthier heart.

Like their cancer-fighting counterparts, foods rich in fiber, folate, and omega-3 fatty acids help to prevent heart disease, stroke, and hypertension. Examples of such foods include nuts, whose unsaturated fat content improves cholesterol levels. Nuts also contain fiber and vitamin E, both of which prevent heart disease and cancer. Oats are another heart-healthy food; a specific fiber in oats helps eliminate cholesterol and lower blood pressure. Fish — especially salmon, herring, anchovies, and sardines — contains omega-3 fatty acids, the much-touted compound that prevents clumping of the blood platelets and in turn prevents heart disease, hypertension, and stroke.

Principle #3

Go ahead, have a glass.

Ever wonder why the French, who eat a diet rich in cheese, meat, and wine, also have one of the lowest rates of coronary heart disease in the world? Numerous studies have shown that red wine, which the French drink a lot of, contains polyphenols that prevent hardening of the arteries. Wine also contains alcohol, which in moderation can prevent heart disease and heart failure. It is important to note that too much alcohol can increase the risk of other diseases, such as cirrhosis of the liver and breast cancer. But in moderation, red wine is a delicious and fun way to keep heart disease at bay.

PRINCIPLE #4

See the clear benefits of eating well.

———————————— ✳ ————————————

Several foods can prevent vision problems and also improve our eyesight. Cold-water fish, such as sardines, cod, mackerel, and tuna, are an excellent source of a fatty acid known as DHA, which helps lubricate eyes and treat macular degeneration. Eggs are rich in cysteine, sulfur, lecithin, and amino acids that protect the lens of the eye from cataract formation. Fruits and vegetables that contain vitamins A, C, E, and beta-carotene, such as carrots and squash, help improve daytime vision, while blueberries and grapes contain anthocyanins, which improve night vision.

Principle #5

Realize that most sugar is not your friend.

There are at least 100 good reasons to avoid eating processed sugars. Among them is the fact that sugar contributes to obesity, tooth decay, diabetes, mood swings, arthritis, decreased vision, heart disease, depression, and the formation of kidney stones. It also has been linked to cancer of the breast, ovaries, prostrate, and rectum. Furthermore, it suppresses the immune system, leaving one vulnerable to colds. If you must eat sugar, do so in its most natural forms. Enjoy the sweetness of fruit, for instance, and try sweetening drinks and desserts with honey. Avoid processed, refined sugars found in soda, cakes, cookies, and ketchup.

Principle #6

Learn the difference between good and bad fat.

Not all fat is created equal. Some fat is so good for you it is necessary to maintain health! The body needs good fats to rebuild body tissue and to absorb vitamins and nutrients. These fats — known as monounsaturated and polysaturated fats — are found in nuts, fish, olives, flaxseed, and tofu. Avoid the class of bad fats that have no nutritional value and can even cause disease and cancer. These include saturated and trans fats, found in meat, dairy, seafood, and packaged foods.

PRINCIPLE #7

Learn healthy cooking techniques.

A meal can start out with healthy ingredients, but the preparation makes the difference between whether you end up eating right or not. There are some people who trick themselves into thinking fried zucchini is a vegetable dish or who douse their plate in so much ranch dressing it defeats the purpose of eating a salad. Make sure you prepare healthy ingredients in healthy ways. Grill, sauté, broil, and bake instead of frying. Remove skin from poultry and other meat. Flavor dishes with broth rather than butter. Use dressings minimally. Use seasonings, not salt. These and other cooking techniques will ensure your healthy ingredients end up as a healthy meal.

Principle #8

Limit your intake of processed and packaged foods.

It would be very difficult to completely cut processed and packaged foods out of our lives. In fact, at one point, the advent of such foods contributed to the increased health of Americans by allowing people to get food no matter the season or where they lived. But today's processed foods tend to be low in nutritional value, containing large amounts of salt, sugar, and fat. They even contain preservatives, chemicals, and fats that endanger our health. So when possible, make foods from scratch or buy them freshly made. You'll be surprised at how quickly most dishes can be homemade, and how much better they taste!

Principle #9

Rethink snack foods.

Everyone gets the munchies now and then. Be sure to have healthy, nutritious snacks on hand for when you get in the mood to munch. Avoid snacks that are high in sugar, salt, and fat, such as chips, cookies, candy, and crackers. Also, build your snacks from different food groups to maximize their nutrition. So, for example, make a snack of apple slices and peanut butter, carrot sticks and hummus, or pita chips and cottage cheese. Snacking can be part of a healthy diet when snacks are nutritious and low-calorie.

PRINCIPLE #10

Eat the most important meal of the day.

——————————— ✳ ———————————

Ever wonder why breakfast has been labeled the most important meal of the day? The answer is simple. When you sleep, you engage in an 8 to 10 hour fast, which causes your metabolism to slow. When your cells do not receive sufficient nutrition immediately following the fast, they fail to function as efficiently. For this reason, people who skip breakfast are more likely to experience fatigue and weight gain. A healthy breakfast can still be had on the go — eat a nutrition bar during your commute, or keep yogurt and cereal at work.

Principle #11

Switch from white to brown.

Grains are an important part of a healthy diet and include foods made from wheat, rice, oats, and cornmeal. Bread, pasta, cereal, and tortillas are examples of grain products. In general, grains come in 2 colors: white or brown, or refined and whole. Refined grains are processed for a longer shelf life, but this removes dietary fiber, iron, and vitamins (and leaves them white). Whole grains, however, are not stripped of their kernel, keeping them brown, nutrient-rich, and lower-calorie. Whole grains also reduce the risk of high cholesterol or blood pressure, diabetes, and certain heart diseases. Choose brown rice, whole wheat pasta and breads, and whole grains for a healthier meal.

Principle #12

Eat the most important meal of the day.

For energy-filled days in which you feel your best, eat 6 small meals instead of 3 big ones. Eating smaller meals more frequently will increase your metabolism and keep insulin levels even through the entire day. Waiting too long between meals teaches your body to revert to starvation mode, which results in storage of fat. This can slow your metabolism and make you feel lethargic.

PRINCIPLE #13

Use food to improve your mood.

Scientific studies have repeatedly found a strong connection between food and mood. Incorporate complex carbohydrates like fruits, vegetables, and whole grains into your diet. Each of these helps maintain levels of serotonin, a mood-elevating chemical in the brain. Nutritionist Susan Kleiner explains the connection between food and mood in the following way. "It's what anti-depressants are all about. These drugs work to elevate serotonin levels or at least keep them from dropping too low. The right foods accomplish the same thing."

Principle #14

Include fish or fish supplements in your diet.

Rotate your menu to feature fish at least once a week. Fish is a leaner, lower-calorie protein than beef, chicken, or pork. Some fishes contain nutrients that improve vision, while others contain compounds that reduce cholesterol and heart disease. Additionally, the omega-3 fatty acids found in certain types of fish (like salmon) are believed to protect the brain from age-related diseases such as Alzheimer's; prevent autoimmune diseases like lupus and arthritis; and even alleviate depression and menstrual cramps. If you dislike fish or are a vegetarian, taking a daily fish-oil supplement in pill form can achieve the same healthful effects.

Exercising and Getting Fit

Author Joey Adams once quipped, "If it weren't for the fact that the TV set and the refrigerator are so far apart, some of us wouldn't get any exercise at all." Adams was remarking on something common to many Americans: a dislike for exercise. Indeed, some of us will do anything to avoid exercise. According to the National Center for Health Statistics, just 3 in 10 Americans exercise regularly. That means 70 percent of the population avoids exercising, despite the plethora of proven health benefits! Physical activity prevents heart disease, stroke, diabetes, cancer, and other conditions that contribute to hundreds of thousands of deaths annually in the United States. Indeed, exercising is one of the most important things you can do to feel better immediately. Exercising also will add to your life span, increasing the years you have available to enjoy yourself.

Many Americans mistakenly believe they are too busy for exercise. However, there is always time to exercise if you build it into your daily routine. Try cutting your lunch break in half and go for a brisk walk after your meal. Or, walk around your neighborhood before or after dinner. Finally, get exercise through the activities already on your to-do list. In fact, everyday chores, if done properly, can substitute for a more formal exercise routine. For example, an hour of washing and drying dishes burns approximately 129 calories; mowing the lawn burns about 200. Get the most out of activities you have to do anyway by incorporating exercise into them.

Finally, realize that exercising always makes you feel better. Studies have shown that engaging in frequent exercise will improve your mood in as little as 2 weeks. When you exercise, your body releases endorphins, which naturally elevate your mood and give you more energy. Your body will become addicted to the natural high that endorphins provide. You will find that the more time you spend being active, the more exercise you will want to do, further serving your goals to feel better and live longer. Follow these simple principles to begin today.

PRINCIPLE #15

Make exercise fun!

———————————— ✳ ————————————

Former Oklahoma Governor David Walters once observed, "An hour of basketball feels like 15 minutes. An hour on a treadmill feels like a weekend in traffic school." Indeed, exercising is unpleasant when you dislike the activity. So choose a form of exercise you enjoy doing! If you hate running on the treadmill, play a sport such as tennis, baseball, or soccer. If you love being in water, join a gym with a lap pool. Other fun ways of getting exercise include taking a ballroom dance class, playing fetch with your dog, or going for a hike. Make your primary source of exercise is also your primary source of fun.

Principle #16

Turn ordinary chores into a fitness routine.

Get the most out of activities you have to do anyway by incorporating exercise into them. Do squats as you fold laundry. Do arm curls with books as you replace them on shelves around your house. Be on the lookout for ways to turn ordinary chores into exercises that count. Even chores themselves can be sources of exercise. An hour of gardening burns approximately 281 calories; vacuuming burns about 246. If you make time to clean your house, you have also just made time to exercise.

Principle #17

Exercise to avoid disease.

Studies repeatedly show that regularly exercising reduces the risk of developing coronary artery disease, diabetes, high blood pressure, high cholesterol, hypertension, obesity, osteoporosis, lipid profiles, mental health, stroke, cancer, and other diseases. Because of its ability to prevent so many illnesses, exercising increases longevity in nearly everyone who practices it, so exercise to make the most of your life. As the English statesman Edward Stanley warned hundreds of years ago, "Those who think they have not time for bodily exercise will sooner or later have to find time for illness."

PRINCIPLE #18

Get a natural high.

Analyst Carol Welch has described exercise in the following way: "Movement is a medicine for creating change in a person's physical, emotional, and mental states." Indeed, when you exercise, you don't merely work your muscles and burn a few calories. You change your body's biochemistry. Exercising causes the body to release endorphins, which naturally elevate your mood and give you more energy. In fact, drugs, including heroin, cocaine, and morphine, all work by releasing endorphins in the body; you can experience a milder, safer, and completely natural high just by exercising. Endorphins leave you feeling great for up to 12 hours after your exercise session.

PRINCIPLE #19

Rise, shine, and exercise.

Author Marsha Doble once joked, "I have to exercise in the morning before my brain figures out what I'm doing." Exercising in the morning is one of the best things you can do for yourself! Studies show that working out first thing in the morning helps to burn more calories from fat due to the way we sleep and wake. Exercising early also means you will release endorphins first thing in the morning, helping you feel alert, energetic, and focused throughout the day. Finally, exercising early means you will be less likely to skip it after a long day.

Principle #20

Take the trial out of errands.

Tired of sweating like a pig when unloading the groceries from the car? Embarrassed by getting winded simply from walking up a flight of stairs? Exercising regularly puts your body in good enough shape to remove these irritations from everyday physical tasks. In addition to building muscles, regular exercise strengthens your cardiovascular system, the system that circulates blood through your heart and blood vessels. When your cardiovascular system is in good shape, it takes more to get you out of breath. In other words, regularly exercising makes other tasks easier and more enjoyable, allowing you to breeze through your day without difficulty.

PRINCIPLE #21

Rev up to wind down.

No one feels their best if they have not gotten a good night's sleep. Exercising for at least 30 minutes can improve the quality and duration of your sleep and also help you fall asleep faster. While exercise wakes you up immediately after doing it, it makes you naturally tired when it is time to go to bed (versus falling asleep from boredom or lethargy). Plus, your body temperature naturally dips about 5 to 6 hours after you exercise, which also helps your body fall asleep. For all these reasons, exercise has been shown to promote a better night's sleep and also reduce insomnia and other sleep disorders.

Principle #22

Realize that when you look your best, you feel your best.

Regular exercise tones muscles, burns fat, and even improves the appearance of skin and hair. Overall, you are sure to look tighter, trimmer, thinner, and more alive as a result of exercising. And everyone knows when a person looks good, they feel tremendous. Looking better results in higher self-esteem, better disposition, and an increased ability to socialize, which can significantly improve your personal and professional life.

GETTING ENOUGH SLEEP

Philosopher Arthur Schopenhauer once remarked, "Sleep is the interest we have to pay on the capital which is called in at death; and the higher the rate of interest and the more regularly it is paid, the further the date of redemption is postponed." Even in the 19th century, Schopenhauer and his contemporaries knew that getting a good night's sleep is essential to extending one's life.

Indeed, getting enough sleep is not only key to living a longer life but living one of higher quality. People who sleep well report higher levels of job satisfaction, mood, better eating habits; and lower levels of marital or familial problems, depression, and illness.

According to the National Sleep Foundation, lack of sleep leads to severe health problems that include chronic fatigue, obesity, high blood pressure, heart disease, suppressed immune system, depression, and shortened life span. Worse, sleep problems and disorders have reached epidemic proportions in the United States: The National Institute of Neurological Disorders and Stroke estimates about 60 million Americans suffer from some sort mild or serious sleep problem. Why are so many Americans having trouble sleeping?

One explanation is the lack of time available to devote to sleep. Studies show that, on average, Americans sleep 6.9 hours a day, which is an hour less than a few decades ago and also an hour less than recommended by doctors. In addition to working more hours and taking less vacation, Americans are increasingly stressed year to year. Especially since the events of September 11, 2001, Americans have reported having fitful nights of sleep during which they worry about the safety of family and friends and whether they will be the victim of a terrorist attack or similar catastrophe.

If you intend to live a healthy and longer life, it is critical you improve your ability to get a good night's sleep. It is no exaggeration to say that sleep is one of the building blocks of life. It is essential for keeping the immune system functioning, and quality sleep has been shown to fight disease and sickness. Sleep is also required to keep the nervous system functioning;

to be able to learn new things; and to function emotionally, mentally, and physically. Last, sleep is essential for cell growth and healing. To extend your life and feel better living it, use the following principles to start sleeping better tonight.

Principle #23

Do not become dependent on sleeping pills.

Sleeping pills are safe when taken temporarily for a specific reason. But they should never be used as a long-term solution to sleep problems. When taken for more than a few weeks, their effect weakens, and they create dependency. Furthermore, the use of sleeping pills over long periods of time can cause "rebound insomnia," an elevated level of insomnia that returns when you stop taking the pills. If you have a history of using sleeping pills and want to stop, look into natural or herbal sleep aids that are phyto-based or contain kava kava. These are mild and non-addicting, but as with all medications, consult your doctor or pharmacist.

PRINCIPLE #24

Never use your bedroom for activities that do not belong there.

In the same way you wouldn't cook food in your bathroom, keep your bedroom reserved for the activities that belong there: sleep and sex. A common mistake many of us make is to bring into the bedroom activities that interfere with our ability to relax. Avoid keeping a television in your bedroom, and skip the temptation to eat, smoke, or drink in bed. Above all, never do work in the bedroom — it is in complete contradiction to everything that room is for.

Principle #25

Avoid stimulants around bedtime.

Most of us realize that a cup of coffee at 9:30 p.m. will interfere with our chances of getting a good night's sleep. But it is just as important to avoid other stimulants, such as nicotine, soda, tea, chocolate, alcohol, spices, red meat, and certain medications, such as diet pills. Avoid consuming these items after 4 p.m. to maximize your chances of a peaceful night's sleep. Trading these indulgences for a good night's sleep will improve your health and well-being in several areas at once.

Principle #26

Keep a regular schedule.

Writer Jessamyn West captured the starkness of insomnia when she wrote, "Sleeplessness is a desert without vegetation or inhabitants." Indeed, those who have experienced sleeplessness know it is extremely frustrating, unsatisfying, and even painful. Increase your ability to sleep by keeping a regular schedule. This will train your biological clock to know when it is supposed to wake or sleep. Keeping a regular schedule is recommended by all sleep clinics to improve the sleep experience. If you can, get your body clock to where you don't need an alarm clock; relying on alarm clocks has been shown to interrupt sleep cycles, which causes a person to feel groggy.

Principle #27

Color yourself to sleep.

Make sure your bedroom is an environment that will facilitate sleep. Decorate it with colors and shapes that are conducive to rest and relaxation. Indeed, color therapy, or phototherapy, is a growing scientific field that has proven that certain colors trigger hormonal responses in humans. For example, the color blue triggers calmness, coolness, and rest. Likewise, indigo has been shown to help the mind enter a meditative state. Choose these shades when decorating your bedroom. Avoid shades of red, which stimulate the appetite, and shades of orange, which put people in a social or festive mood.

Principle #28

Create a bedtime routine.

Philosopher Friedrich Nietzsche once remarked, "Sleeping is no mean art: for its sake one must stay awake all day." In other words, sleeping is something many of us may have to work for! To make your work easier, create a bedtime routine. Doing so will signal to both your mind and body that the time to sleep is near. Your routine should be tailored to activities, sights, and sounds that relax you. Listen to ambient music; light a candle; read something that bores you; practice deep breathing exercises. No matter what your bedtime routine consists of, stick to it every night, even on weekends..

Principle #29

Don't take your stress to bed with you.

According to the Better Sleep Council's annual stress and sleep survey, 65 percent of Americans lose sleep because of stress. It is difficult to shelve our deepest fears, concerns, and worries when it's time to go to bed, but critically important. To avoid going to bed stressed, spend the hours before bedtime doing relaxing activities that take your mind off your problems. Read a chatty magazine or an engaging novel, or play solitaire on the computer. The end of the night is never a good time to look at work, check email, or pay bills, which are all key causes of stress.

Principle #30

Don't get too much sleep.

To those who have trouble sleeping, it may seem like you'd want to catch all the zzz's you can. But research has shown that adults need a maximum of 8 hours of sleep a night in order to feel alert and awake the next day. Sleeping beyond 8 hours can actually make you groggier and more lethargic throughout your day. So, unless you are catching up from jet lag or a rare all-nighter, don't let yourself sleep your way to grogginess.

PRINCIPLE #31

Don't force it.

Author C.S. Lewis once noted, "Many things — such as loving, going to sleep, or behaving unaffectedly — are done worst when we try hardest to do them." Indeed, pushing yourself to go to sleep almost never works; instead it tends to result in hours of staring at the crack in the ceiling. If you can't fall asleep within 30 minutes of initially trying, give up. It is better to do something else for an hour to tire yourself out than to lie in bed with insomnia.

Principle #32

If you have a sleep disorder, see a doctor.

According to the National Institute of Neurological Disorders and Stroke, about 40 million people in the U.S. suffer from chronic long-term sleep disorders each year. If you have serious and continued trouble sleeping, see a health specialist; you may have one of more than 70 sleep disorders, which include sleep apnea (stoppages in breathing during sleep, characterized by excessive snoring), insomnia, and sleepwalking. In addition to seeing a doctor, contact sleep clinics in your area; you may be able to take part in a study on sleep disorders in exchange for free or discounted medical care.

TAKING TIME TO RELAX AND MEDITATE

It's hard to believe that pop star Madonna will be 50 years old. She looks like she could easily be in her mid-30s. And in fact, she continues to look better as she gets older. Her secret? She eats a healthy diet and regularly practices yoga and meditation. Something Madonna learned early on is that aging gracefully must be approached holistically and from the inside out. Meditation is an excellent way to do this. Yoga, Tai Chi, deep breathing, and sitting quietly are all forms of meditation you should begin learning in order to feel better and live longer.

Studies repeatedly show that meditation improves practitioners' appearance, mindset, physical health, and general sense of well-being. Meditation can be a quick and easy way to feel less stressed out. When practiced regularly, meditation can also induce a deeper sense of relaxation, which must be achieved to balance our increasingly fast-paced lifestyles. Indeed, in a world filled with stressors such as constant noise, financial difficulties, extended work hours, and long commutes it is no wonder many of us find it so difficult to relax.

A wonderful aspect of meditation is that it can be done easily, quickly, inexpensively, and almost anywhere. Just practicing for 5 minutes can unleash its healing and restorative effects. Meditation instantly relaxes by increasing blood flow and slowing the heart rate while decreasing muscle tension and headaches. Meditation also reduces anxiety attacks by lowering the levels of lactic acid in the blood. High levels of lactic acid have been proven to lead to increased anxiety. Of course, meditation alone won't do the trick — you must also avoid foods that increase lactic acid in the blood, which include chocolate, refined sugar, alcohol, wheat, salt, commercial salad dressings, ketchup, mustard, coffee, black tea, and red meat. Combining meditation with a high-nutrient diet that includes lots of green vegetables, brown rice, whole grains, seeds and nuts, fruits, poultry, fish, olive oil, and flax seeds or oil can help relieve stress.

Even though it may not feel like it, the most important time to relax is when you feel you cannot afford to do so. As journalist Sydney J. Harris reminds us, "The time to relax is when you don't have time for it." Be sure to consult the following simple principles the next time you feel overwhelmed and find it difficult to relax. You will discover quick tips for instant relief that can be easily incorporated into your daily life.

Principle #33

Learn how to breathe.

You have been taking breaths since the moment you were born, but have you ever considered that after all this time you don't know how to properly do it? Most of us breathe too shallow to harness the relaxing and meditative benefits of breathing. Breathing properly requires you to deeply inhale using your diaphragm, not your chest. This moves air through your whole respiratory system, not just your upper lungs. Inhale for a count of 5. Hold your breath briefly, then slowly exhale through your mouth for another count of 5. Repeat several times. Carve 5 minutes out of every day to focus on concentrated breathing to maximize relaxation.

PRINCIPLE #34

Practice yoga to unwind.

The health benefits of yoga are far-reaching and varied. Yoga increases flexibility, which increases the range of motion in your joints. It also acts as strength-training since many of the poses are weight-bearing and held for long lengths of time. Yoga also helps to define and sculpt muscles, which will improve your physique. Regular yoga practice forces you to breathe deeply, thus increasing the blood flow and oxygen to your limbs and organs. All of these physical benefits lead to a sense of calm and relaxation. Yoga helps to alleviate stress and brings a sense of control and mindfulness to everyday activities.

Principle #35

Choose a mantra that fits your personality.

A mantra is a sound you make that creates a vibration that helps you concentrate on the moment. It is a tool used during meditation. Tsangsar Tulku Rinpoche defined the 6-syllable mantra used in many Buddhist traditions: Om (meditation or bliss), Ma (patience), Ni (discipline), Pad (wisdom), Me (generosity), and Hum (diligence). You may want to choose just one that speaks most to your personality. Or, hum the chants all together, saying, "Om Mani Padme Hum." You should chant in a droning tone that causes you to feel relaxed yet alert and focused.

Principle #36

Carry a set of beads.

— ❋ —

Keep a set of beads to use for quick and subtle meditations. Beads can be carried in the form of rosaries, Buddhist prayer beads (malas), or even just a cheap string with plastic beads. Your beads should be accessible to you at all times, while in your car, at work, or in your home. When you feel stressed, pick up your beads, touch each of them, and say an affirmation or prayer. If you're on an airplane and feeling anxious, your affirmation might be, "I am safe." Repeat the same affirmation or prayer as you move your fingers over the beads. Continue to do so until you feel more relaxed.

Principle #37

Use guided imagery to relax.

Guided imagery is a relaxation technique in which you listen to descriptions of calming images. Enlist the help of a therapist or friend to describe these images, or make a recording of your own voice. An example of guided imagery is to imagine yourself in the center of a triangle. Picture the triangle filling with cool, blue light. The combination of the image along with it being delivered in a soothing tone has been shown to reduce anxiety up to 65 percent and decrease pain and reduce stress within minutes. It is so relaxing, in fact, that people are warned not to listen to guided imagery recordings while driving.

Principle #38

Practice walking meditation.

Walking meditation is a great way for beginners to practice meditation. One reason meditating while in motion is easier for people is because sitting in the lotus position can be challenging. It is also difficult to shut out distractions. Walking meditation, on the other hand, allows you to focus on the movements of your body. As Buddhism expert Charles MacInerny explains, "Be mindful of your walking, make each step a gesture, so that you move in a state of grace, and each footprint is an impression of the peace and love you feel for the universe. Walk with slow, small, deliberate, balanced, graceful footsteps."

Principle #39

Take a vacation using journey meditation.

Journey meditation is a great way to get an afternoon pick-me-up or to unwind after a long day at work. It is a type of meditation that integrates deep breathing with visualization exercises and will leave you feeling refreshed and recharged. Sit in a comfortable position and think of a peaceful place. A quiet beach is an ideal mental destination. Picture yourself resting on warm white sand. Feel the soothing sun warming your skin. Hear waves crash against the sand and then retreat. Listen to seagulls cry and to the low moan of a ship horn. Be specific and detailed, and practice twice a day.

Principle #40

Tai Chi your way to a calmer state.

Tai Chi first originated 2,000 years ago in China as a form of self-defense and has evolved into an elegant form of exercise. It is very popular internationally due to its ability to reduce stress, give greater balance, and increase flexibility. Studies show that older adults benefit greatly from Tai Chi practice because it reduces the risk of falling. Tai Chi movements are low-impact and therefore appropriate for all fitness levels. Find a Tai Chi center or instructor in your community to take part in this age-old relaxing practice.

Principle #41

Incorporate positive affirmations into your daily routine.

Saying positive affirmations or statements to yourself is an excellent way to both relax and develop confidence. Positive thinking does not come naturally to most of us but is essential for reprogramming negative thoughts and achieving relaxation. Instead of telling yourself, "I am too fat," think, "I am beautiful and working toward my goal weight." Not only will affirming the positive relax you, it will also extend your life; a recent study by Mayo Clinic researchers found that people who think positively live 19 percent longer than those who do not.

Principle #42

Relax yourself with ambient music.

Put yourself in a calm, relaxed zone by listening to low, ambient sounds or music. Ambient simply means "of the environment." Some people respond to simple drumbeats with flutes, while others find the sound of waves crashing or crickets to be relaxing. Musician Brian Eno states, "Ambient music must be able to accommodate many levels of listening attention without enforcing one in particular; it must be as ignorable as it is interesting." Combining ambient sounds with deep breathing exercises can put you into a deep state of relaxation that allows your mind and body to de-stress and recharge.

Finding Ways to Be Happy

For centuries, humans have spent gobs of money, time, and energy attempting to discover the fountain of youth, the Holy Grail, or fabled elixirs that would extend or result in eternal life. Indeed, discovering a way to live longer has been the pursuit of explorers, apothecaries, and religious aficionados. But anyone who has ever pursued a longer life would be surprised to discover they already carry the keys to longevity within them: their happiness.

It seems incredible, but becoming a happier person actually helps you live a longer life. This has been confirmed by several prominent studies. In one, researchers at Yale University found that optimists live 7½ years longer than those who are gloomy or depressed. The study also found that simply being a happy person adds, on average, 9 years to one's life. Another study reported in the British paper *The Daily Mail* found that having lots of friends, living in the countryside, and being in a happy marriage can add up to 20 years to a person's life. Together, these and other studies show that achieving happiness by making just a few small changes to your lifestyle, mentality, and outlook can delay death for years.

However, most Americans are far from discovering the life-giving properties of happiness. In fact, the U.S. reports the lowest level of happiness of any industrialized country. According to reporter John Lanchester in an article from The New Yorker magazine, "Looking at the data from all over the world, it is clear that, instead of getting happier as they become better off, people get stuck on a 'hedonic treadmill': their expectations rise at the same pace as their incomes, and the happiness they seek remains constantly just out of reach." In addition to being stuck on this treadmill, the happiness of many is stalled by our increasingly materialistic and expensive culture. Financial strain is the number one reason people cite for why they are unable to be happy. Body image is a close second. According to BBC News, "More than 70 percent of women had made serious attempts to diet in the last year and 58 percent had 'disordered' eating patterns." Too many of us make ourselves miserable trying to look a certain way and damage our prospects for long life in the process.

If you want to live longer, it is essential that you learn to be a happier person. The best thing about happiness is that there exists an infinite supply. We need only tap into the various sources within us to start living a happier life today. The following principles will help you find these sources within yourself and give you ideas for how to bring more joy into your life.

Principle #43

Accept who you are.

———————————— ❊ ————————————

George Orwell wrote, "Happiness can exist only in acceptance." If you long to be happier, you must work to accept who you are. You must never hold against yourself the things you cannot change — your family, ethnicity, religion, physical, or emotional shortcomings. Learn to see these qualities as part and parcel of a perfectly imperfect you. In accepting who you are, isolate those parts of yourself that can be improved upon (such as furthering your education, losing weight, or becoming more organized). Work toward your goals by understanding the difference between the aspects of your life that can and cannot be changed.

Principle #44

Define your faith and values.

Think of the happiest person you know. If you were to ask his secret, he would probably tell you his happiness stems from having faith. Indeed, believing in something larger than you will help put setbacks into perspective and can even extend your life. Indeed, this was the conclusion of 42 studies whose results were published together in Health Psychology. The studies found that those who regularly attend a house of worship live significantly longer than those who do not.

Principle #45

Learn to forgive.

Learning to forgive is an excellent way to become a happier person. Life is difficult enough; adding years of collected resentments will drag you down, making you unhappy, and, consequently, unhealthy. When you forgive someone who wronged you, you release resentment that unhealthily burdened you. This does not mean that you must forget the event. It simply means you set yourself free from the negative feelings associated with the person who wronged you. It was for this reason that theology professor Lewis B. Smedes wrote, "To forgive is to set a prisoner free and discover that the prisoner was you."

Principle #46

Focus on what is right in your life.

An old Swedish proverb states, "Worry often gives small things a big shadow." Indeed, we make mountains out of molehills by needlessly obsessing over things that are imperfect in our lives. Resist the urge to fixate on what you want to change about yourself or your circumstances. Instead, focus on what is working in your life, and channel your energy into those areas. Nurturing the good parts of life allows them to flourish and makes you feel like a happier person.

Principle #47

Smile often — even when you don't feel like it.

Even when you don't mean it, a smile can make you feel happier. Smiling releases endorphins, natural pain killers produced by the brain. In addition, put positive thinking behind your smile; a 2005 study by the Wake Forest University Baptist Medical Center found that thinking positively actually helps people overcome pain. In fact, Dr. Tetsuo Koyama, the lead author of the study, said, "Positive expectations produced about a 28 percent decrease in pain ratings — equal to a shot of morphine." So smile — it is a simple way to change the way you feel from the outside in.

Principle #48

Become aware of the happiness you experience every day.

— ✳ —

Our overall happiness is a product of our daily experiences. We all have positive experiences every day but some pay less attention to them than others. For 1 week, keep a list of experiences that made you feel happy. No enjoyment is too small to record. For example, take note if you tried a delicious new food or found a way to save $15 on your cable bill. At the end of the week, notice how many little joys life throws at you, and be sure to repeat them to find your way to happiness.

Principle #49

Learn to love your appearance.

According to a poll of 380,000 citizens of more than 225 countries, just 35 percent of people enjoy the view when they look in the mirror. That means when 65 percent of the world's population looks in the mirror, they are disappointed! Feel happier every day by loving the way you look. Stare in the mirror and find something about yourself that pleases you. Say, "I have beautiful skin," or "I like the way this color looks on me." After a while, you will learn to love the whole image — and nothing helps a person feel happier than feeling good about the way they look.

Principle #50

Say goodbye to the green-eyed monster.

————————— ✳ —————————

Jealousy is universally recognized as one of the ugliest human emotions. People who use jealousy as their primary way of dealing with others suffer from severe insecurity and unhappiness. If you are a jealous person, you are likely trapped by anger, fear, hatred, and loneliness. It is simply not possible to be happy when consumed by these feelings. The author William Penn once insightfully noted, "The jealous are troublesome to others, but a torment to themselves." Don't torture yourself with feelings of jealousy. Everyone gets jealous now and then, but if you want to be happy, you must eliminate jealousy from your life.

PRINCIPLE #51

Never compare your life with another.

───────────── ✳ ─────────────

Comparing your life to another person's is like comparing apples and bananas or dogs and cats. Because everyone is so different, you are bound to come up short in some area. Interestingly, siblings especially tend to compare their lives in detrimental ways. A study published in the Journal of Family Communication found that 52 percent of all people experience a jealousy incident within their family. Comparing your life with family members and others will cause you to feel unnecessarily unhappy. Avoid this common pitfall, and find happiness in comparing yourself only to your own past and present.

Principle #52

Learn anger-management skills.

It is said that for every minute you are angry, you lose 60 seconds of happiness. Everyone gets angry sometimes, but studies show that people who successfully manage their anger consistently report low incidents of depression and unhappiness. To be like them, get a handle on your anger. Deal with small annoyances as they come rather than waiting until you explode with rage. When you feel anger coming on, take deep breaths. Use logic, rationality, and facts to win arguments, not anger. Focusing your energy on life's challenges effectively rather than angrily will make you a happier person, which is critical for living a longer, healthier life.

Principle #53

Experience the joy of giving.

The increasingly self-absorbed nature of our culture causes many of us to feel lonely and disconnected from one another. People who give to charity or volunteer, on the other hand, feel valued and needed. Feeling generous helps us to be happy, purposeful, and complete. To experience the joy of giving, investigate charities in your area. Perhaps you can serve meals at a church once a month, help build homes, or donate money to a children's group organizing a field trip. Giving your time and money to a worthy cause helps put your own problems in perspective, involves you in a community, and enhances your sense of happiness.

Principle #54

Quit smoking right now.

Introducing the latest good reason to quit smoking: It is a surefire way to become a happier person. Former smokers consistently testify that they are happier than when they smoked. In fact, a poll taken by the American Cancer Society found that 85 percent of former smokers wished they had quit at least 5 years earlier than they did. Not only do their clothes, hair, and breath no longer smell of cigarettes, but they are no longer socially isolated for their habit. Furthermore, those who do not smoke tend to exercise more, and exercising releases endorphins, which naturally elevate your mood.

Principle #55

Laugh out loud!

Studies show that laughter reduces stress, lowers blood pressure, elevates mood, boosts the immune system, improves brain functioning, increases oxygen in the blood, fosters connection with others, and makes you feel good all over. Children in nursery school laugh approximately 300 times a day, while adults laugh, at most, only 17 times per day. So incorporate a good chuckle into your day to make sure you are getting the health benefits that happiness has to offer.

PRINCIPLE #56

Develop a sense of purpose.

Achieving happiness goes hand in hand with developing a strong sense of purpose. The state of mind you have when absorbed in the accomplishment of a goal is an engaged, satisfied state. Those who have learned to develop a sense of purpose are the most likely to be happy and healthy. Happiness researcher Martin Seligman writes that developing a sense of purpose can increase a person's happiness over time. "It's about being in the flow, completely absorbed by your work, the pursuit of your goals, the people you love, and your leisure activities," says Seligman.

Principle #57

Know that you are responsible for your own happiness.

Never rely on your relationships as the primary source of your happiness. If you put that responsibility onto others, they will let you down over and over again. Your happiness is simply not something that others can provide. Relationships should enhance your happiness, not serve as its sole source. In truth, you are the only one who is able to be responsible for your happiness. Depending on any one person to make you happy will leave you feeling disappointed and unfulfilled. Learn to find things within yourself that make you truly happy.

Principle #58

Maintain a positive outlook.

---------- ❋ ----------

The benefits of positive thinking are plentiful. Researchers have concluded that people who think positively live longer and healthier lives than those who think pessimistically. Some health benefits of positive thinking are reduced stress, resistance to colds, easier breathing, stable heart rate, and lower blood pressure. Studies also show that positive thinkers tend to make healthier choices, such as eating well and avoiding excess alcohol or drugs. Therefore, thinking positively is critical to achieving health and happiness. There is no more-powerful tool available to a person than his thoughts. As Abraham Lincoln once said, "Most folks are about as happy as they make up their minds to be."

PRINCIPLE #59

Boost your self-esteem.

Saturday Night Live character Stuart Smalley used to close his sketch with, "I am good enough, I am smart enough, and gosh darn it, people like me." Though meant to be funny, Smalley's instinct to boost his ego is correct. You probably spend time each day telling yourself what you should have done, what you could have done better, or what you find unsatisfying about yourself. These messages will stall your happiness. Become a happier person by changing the way you talk to yourself. Within a few weeks of saying good things about yourself, you will notice you feel much happier.

Principle #60

Take care of yourself.

If your body is not happy, your mind won't be either. To develop a happy outlook, make sure to practice basic self-care, even when stretched thin. Get outdoors every day for at least 30 minutes. The fresh air and exercise will clear your head and release endorphins, which will give you a natural high. Make healthy choices when you eat. Eating foods that nourish your body (greens, lean protein, whole grains) will give you energy to carry you through your day. Practicing regular self-care is a natural way to elevate your mood.

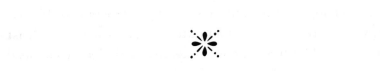

Keeping Yourself Hydrated

"Water, thou hast no taste, no color, no odor; canst not be defined, art relished while ever mysterious. Not necessary to life, but rather life itself, thou fillest us with a gratification that exceeds the delight of the senses." French author Antoine de Saint-Exupery wrote this ode to water in his 1939 book, From Wind, Sand and Stars. Saint-Exupery put into words what countless others have come to recognize: Water is essential to life, and increasing your consumption can dramatically improve the way you feel and even extend your life span.

To appreciate how critical water is for your survival, consider that the human body is made up of about 60 to 70 percent water. The skin, the body's largest organ, is 90 percent water! Blood is composed of about 82 percent water, while muscles and the brain are constituted by 75 percent water. Even bones are part water — 25 percent. Water is clearly an integral part of every piece of your body, it depends on your intake of water to keep your physiological systems running properly.

But every day, we lose water through natural and necessary functions such as breathing, perspiring, urinating, and eliminating waste. Other activities, such as exercising, walking, straining, swimming, and living in dry or high altitude climates, further draw moisture from our bodies. Finally, many of the foods and drinks we consume — such as coffee, soda, and alcohol — are terrifically dehydrating, causing our bodies to lose even more fluids.

Some of the many advantages to staying well hydrated include having more energ, feeling more focused, reducing your risk of cancer, losing weight, avoiding the uncomfortable and health-hazardous symptoms of dehydration, and keeping your skin fresh for a younger look. To get these advantages, employ the following simple principles to keep your body hydrated — in doing so, you will put yourself on the path to feeling better and living longer.

Principle #61

Become familiar with the life-giving properties of water.

Nobel Prize winner Albert Szent-Gyorgyi once said, "Water is life's matter and matrix, mother and medium. There is no life without water." Indeed, humans can survive for up to 2 months without food but succumb in a week without water. Water is essential for every biological function. It removes waste products from the body and facilitates chemical reactions that jumpstart digestion, metabolism, and respiration. It carries nutrients and oxygen to the cells through the blood and helps cool the body. There is a reason that 60 to 70 percent of the body is comprised of water — it truly is the building block of life.

PRINCIPLE #62

Use water to lose weight.

Drinking more water will help you lose weight in 3 ways. First, you will avoid dehydration, which studies show slows metabolism — the body's fat-burning process — by as much as 3 percent. Second, drinking water helps you eat less by causing you to feel fuller. A University of Washington study found 1 glass of water curbed midnight hunger pangs in almost 100 percent of dieters. Finally, drinking water helps your body stay toned. Says Dr. Howard Flaks, an obesity specialist, "By not drinking enough water, many people incur excess body fat, [and] poor muscle tone and size." Plus, losing weight increases life span by helping you avoid illnesses such as diabetes.

Principle #63

Think outside the bottle.

Bottled water sells well, but don't assume it is any purer than tap water. In a recent study, the Natural Resources Defense Council found that ⅓ of all bottled waters contain bacteria or chemicals that exceed state purity standards. Furthermore, bottled water creates waste — beverage industry consultant R. W. Beck, Inc. estimates that only 12 percent of all water bottles are recycled, while 40 million are thrown away every day. Instead of bottled water, install a water filter onto your tap, or buy a refrigerator with a built-in filter. For water on the go, refill a polyurethane bottle, found at outdoors stores.

Principle #64

Defy cancer with water.

With cancer rates at an all-time high, you want to do everything you can to avoid developing this awful disease in its myriad forms. Increasing your water intake can help you do that. Studies have shown that drinking at least 5 glasses of water a day can decrease the risk of colon cancer by 45 percent, decrease the risk of developing bladder cancer by 50 percent, and decrease the risk of developing breast cancer by a whopping 79 percent.

PRINCIPLE #65

Get an energy boost.

Looking for an energy drink? Choose water. Studies show that lack of water is the number one cause of daytime fatigue. In fact, just a 2 percent drop in the body's water supply can trigger short-term memory problems and cause you to have difficulty focusing. Ironically, sugary sport drinks that purport to increase energy do quite the opposite — they give you a temporary boost that is usually followed by a crash. For a true energy boost and improved concentration, drink water. Perhaps the great American writer Henry David Thoreau was thinking of water's energizing properties when he wrote, "I believe that water is the only drink for a wise man."

Principle #66

Don't wait to get thirsty.

Never use your thirst as a guide for when to drink more water. By the time you get around to feeling thirsty, your body has already started to dehydrate. Dehydration causes fatigue, headache, muscle weakness, dizziness, and slows physiological processes including metabolism, respiration, and digestion. Be aware that dehydration is not caused by sun exposure or physical activity alone. The body's regular processes consume water at an incredible rate — it is even possible to lose a pint of water each day simply by exhaling! What's more, as we age, our bodies become less able to sense dehydration, making thirst an even poorer indication of when we need water.

Principle #67

Discover the fountain of youth.

— ※ —

We all know that swimming in water for too long wrinkles our skin. But water has the opposite effect when we ingest it. Indeed, staying hydrated is key to keep skin looking young and wrinkle-free. The skin — the body's largest organ — is 90 percent water. When it becomes dry, it loses elasticity, which contributes to wrinkles, blemishes, and other defects. Drinking water stimulates the circulation of body fluids such as blood, giving us a rosy complexion. It also clears toxins from the body, which are a cause of pimples. To defy age and keep wrinkles at bay, hydrate your skin from the inside out.

Principle #68

Hydrate according to your climate.

No matter where you live, drinking enough water will help you feel your best. But people living in dry areas, such as the Southwest, need to drink even more than those living in humid climates. Dry climates cause the body to excessively perspire, which draws out moisture at an increased rate. Furthermore, those who live at high altitude (more than 8,000 feet) may use up their body's water reserves faster than others. High altitude triggers increased urination and rapid breathing, which taps the body's fluid reserves. You can tell if you are getting enough water by how often you urinate and whether your urine is darkly colored.

PRINCIPLE #69

Replace soda with water.

———————— ✳ ————————

Soda contributes to weight gain, skin defects, bone density problems, and many other health issues. Sodas contain some of the strongest acids available on the market, such as phosphoric acid. This acid is so deadly that it can dissolve metals (try leaving a penny in a glass of cola overnight!). When inside your body, these acids erode tooth enamel and cause a host of other problems. Most Americans have no idea how bad soda is for them; this is why they continue to drink more than 13 billion gallons every year. Be among the first to feel better and live longer by eliminating soda from your diet.

Principle #70

Hydrate beyond the glass.

You don't need to rely only on what you drink to meet your daily water needs. You can get a significant portion from food. On average, food provides about 20 percent of total water intake, while the remaining 80 percent comes from water and beverages of all kinds. You can increase this amount by eating foods that contain a lot of water. For example, many fruits and vegetables — such as watermelon, celery, tomatoes, and cucumbers — are more than 90 percent water. Milk, broth-based soups, and unsweetened, natural fruit juice are also comprised mostly of water and can help you meet your hydration goals.

Principle #71

Get your 8-a-day the fun way.

─────────────────────────── ❊ ───────────────────────────

There are several ways to make increasing your water intake a delicious and enjoyable experience. Keep a pitcher of cool, filtered water in the fridge. Add lemon, lime, or orange slices for a refreshing twist. In your home, drink water from a wine glass to imitate the casual luxury of dining out. On hot days, suck on ice cubes, or make juice pops from unsweetened, natural fruit juice. Most important, have water on your person at all times so hydrating is easy. Carry a polyurethane jug or other water bottle with you at work, while shopping, and at the gym.

Maintaining a Healthy Heart

In 1978, at Baylor College of Medicine, Dr. Dean Ornish conducted studies on patients with coronary heart disease. He found that within a surprisingly short period, the patients who ate a low-fat vegetarian diet and practiced stress-reduction activities had lower cholesterol and blood pressure than those who did not. They also had increased blood flow to the heart and experienced less chest pain. Ornish found that such lifestyle changes not only prevent heart disease but can actually reverse it. Now an author, physician, and founder of the Preventive Medicine Research Institute, Dr. Ornish has created a program to control coronary artery disease based on diet, exercise, smoking cessation, and meditation or stress-reduction activities.

Ornish's program has yet to reach the masses, however, and so Americans continue to suffer from heart disease. In fact, heart-disease rates in America have reached epidemic proportions;

according to the American Heart Association, 1 out of 3 American adults have one or more types of cardiovascular disease. In some cases, the traits for heart disease are inherited. But more often than not, heart disease is caused by obesity, lack of exercise, high levels of stress, and engaging in vices that harm the heart, such as smoking.

The important thing to realize from this information is that you have control over 4 of the 5 factors that go into maintaining a healthy heart: diet, exercise, stress reduction, and the vices you allow yourself. It may seem overwhelming to consider overhauling your lifestyle, but even small changes help. You must take all opportunities to make these small changes, such as deciding to breathe deeply to calm yourself in stressful situations and ordering a side salad instead of fries. Remember that each time you don't eat something you shouldn't, your heart has time to heal and become stronger. Practicing these simple principles will help your heart strengthen over time, enabling you to lead a longer and more comfortable life.

PRINCIPLE #72

Eat a more vegetarian diet.

Eating a more plant-based diet is perhaps the single most important thing you can do to maintain a healthy heart. Avoid animal products, as their high fats are bad for your heart. In fact, studies show that diets high in dairy products result in clogged arteries, high cholesterol, and a slower metabolism. According to the American Heart Association, vegetarians have "a lower risk of obesity, coronary heart disease, high blood pressure, diabetes mellitus, and some forms of cancer." The AHA recommends getting your protein from lean sources such as soy, tofu, legumes, and fish that have heart-friendly omega-3 fatty acids.

PRINCIPLE #73

Trade in your apple for a pear.

─────────────── ✳ ───────────────

Carrying excess weight around your stomach is a major indicator for future heart disease. So, look in the mirror. Do you resemble an apple or a pear? If you look more like a Fuji than a Bartlett, it's time to work off your middle fat reserve. According to the Johns Hopkins Ciccarone Center for the Prevention of Heart Disease, "People whose fat collects around the waist — the classic apple shape — are at higher risk of heart disease than their pear-shaped counterparts, whose weight collects around the hips." Decrease your middle mass by walking, jogging, swimming, and eating a diet high in fiber and low in fat.

Principle #74

Take your heart for a walk.

It is no wonder that heart disease is the leading cause of death in the U.S. when you consider that 1 in 4 Americans lives a completely sedentary lifestyle. According to the National Heart, Lung, and Blood Institute, to avoid heart disease you should engage in at least 30 minutes of moderate physical activity most days of the week; for maximum heart benefits, exercise 7 days a week. Remember that exercise lowers blood pressure, improves circulation and metabolism, and also boosts energy.

Principle #75

Treat your heart like it is an infant.

---* ---

Pretend your heart is an infant. How would you care for it? Would you give an infant alcohol, cigarettes, or drugs? Of course not! The next time you are tempted to go on a drinking binge, imagine you are poisoning your infant child. Drinking heavily may cause alcohol poisoning, which can result in sudden cardiac death. Also, keep in mind that stimulants such as amphetamines have health effects that include inducing dangerously fast heart rates and high blood pressure — which can also lead to sudden death.

Principle #76

Breathe air, not smoke.

Even though smoking is the most preventable cause of death in the U.S., it accounts for nearly 440,000 of the more than 2.4 million deaths each year. According to the American Heart Association, smokers are at high risk for fatty buildups in their arteries. Other studies indicate that smoking is a direct cause of coronary heart disease, which leads to heart attack. For your heart's sake, quit smoking immediately. By quitting now, you give your body more time to reverse the effects smoking has had on it. So step outside, take a deep breath, and feel the healing begin as you fill your lungs with oxygen-rich air.

PRINCIPLE #77

"Trans-form" your diet.

Most Americans eat heaping portions of animal-based diets that are high in fat, particularly in trans fats. Trans fats are solid fats that are artificially produced by heating liquid vegetable oils in the presence of metal catalysts and hydrogen. According to a Harvard School of Public Health study, "Approximately 30,000 premature coronary heart disease deaths annually could be attributable to consumption of trans fatty acids." Trans fat is found in the oils used to cook fast food, especially in french fries. Baked goods that are sold commercially also often use trans fats as a preservative.

Principle #78

Engage in stress-relieving activities.

Left unmanaged, stress leads to skipped or extra heart beats, coronary artery disease, and high blood pressure. Since it is unrealistic to avoid stress all together, it is necessary to manage it. Stress management expert Elizabeth Scott recommends using the Karate Breathing Method, which takes between 3 and 10 minutes to produce relaxation. This method requires you to sit or kneel and inhale deeply through your nose. Exhale all of the air in your lungs out through your mouth. The trick to this type of breathing is to let your abdomen expand and contract, rather than moving your shoulders up and down.

Principle #79

Shape your lifestyle to fit inside your genes.

Since heart problems tend to be hereditary, it is important to know your family's heart history. For instance, when it comes to cholesterol, genetics tend to determine how bad your problem will be, what you are able to eat, and whether you will need to take medication to lower your cholesterol. While some people are genetically predisposed to low cholesterol, others cannot even consume 1 teaspoon of butter without experiencing a rise in their cholesterol levels. Therefore, find out your predisposition to heart troubles so you can tackle them most efficiently.

PRINCIPLE #80

Express your emotions.

———————————————— ✳ ————————————————

Learning to express your emotions can truly be a matter of life and death. Many of us bottle our anger and sadness, which leads to depression. Take heed, though, as a recent study published in Psychotherapy and Psychosomatics found that one's inability to express emotions is linked to coronary heart disease. Further studies indicate that learning to cope with anger, sadness, and depression can reduce the damage stress wreaks on the heart. In this way, learning to healthily express anger can extend your life span.

PRINCIPLE #81

Love your heart to life.

❋

An often overlooked cause of heart disease is loneliness. In fact, studies show that caring about others and having confidantes has important health benefits. A study by Case Western Reserve University found that married men who answered "yes" when asked, "Does your wife show you her love?" had significantly less chest pain. In another study by Yale University, those who felt loved and supported "had substantially less blockage in their coronary arteries." So, for the good of your heart, if you are feeling lonely, make efforts to enjoy real and satisfying connections with others.

PRINCIPLE #82

Keep bad cholesterol under control with good food choices.

You have control over the cholesterol your body produces after eating. In fact, 25 percent of your total cholesterol is made as your body digests food. A diet high in saturated or trans fats causes the body to produce too much LDL, or "bad" cholesterol. According to the American Heart Association, when LDL cholesterol builds up in the blood it forms "a thick, hard deposit that can narrow the arteries and make them less flexible." This condition, known as atherosclerosis, greatly increases your risk for heart attack and stroke. You can, however, limit your cholesterol numbers through your dietary choices.

MAINTAINING HEALTHY BONES

When asked to name a few of the living tissues of their body, most people will name muscles or organs. Few, however, realize that their bones are living tissues. Indeed, the human skeletal system is a tissue that, like a muscle, can be made strong or weak depending on how you treat it. And in order to feel better and live a longer life, you must make it a priority to develop strong bones as early as possible.

Indeed, a major physical aspect of aging is the loss of bone density. Bone density refers to how much bone mineral is packed into a particular segment of bone — the more minerals, the healthier and stronger the bone. Loss of bone density results in the development of the bone disease osteoporosis, which causes bones to become more fragile and likely to break. Having weak bones puts you at risk for fractures and breaks, which, as you age, are more difficult to recover from. In fact, Dr. John Abramson says, "Because 9 out of 10 hip fractures result from falls, engaging in activities that increase strength and balance helps decrease the risk. Strength training is one of the best ways to increase bone density in the spine naturally and prevent falls." Humans begin losing bone density at around age 35, though how much and how rapidly they lose it depends on a number of factors, including diet, exercise, lifestyle, and family history.

Though both women and men are vulnerable to osteoporosis, postmenopausal women are particularly at risk. Due to hormonal changes in the postmenopausal body, a woman can lose up to 20 percent of her bone mass in just 5 to 10 years. Osteoporosis can be devastating. It is estimated that more than half of all women, and 1 in 3 men, will develop bone fractures due to osteoporosis. By the time they are 70, more than 20 percent of all women will have been hospitalized from a fracture or break due to osteoporosis. Osteoporosis also causes loss of height, pain, and development of a back hump, often referred to as a "dowager's hump."

Your risk of developing osteoporosis can be minimized, however, by following the simple principles in this chapter for maintaining healthy bones.

Principle #83

Jump around!

Researchers at the Bone Research Laboratory at Oregon State University advise people who are strong enough to jump to counteract bone density loss. Jumping is an excellent, simple, and fast way to add bone mass at the hip and increase agility. Three times a week, on a flat, even surface, jump up as high as you can. Be sure to slightly bend your knees and land on flat feet. Jump near a sturdy object you can hold on to in case of a fall, such as a chair or desk. Start with 10 to 30 jumps a session and, as you get stronger, aim for 40 to 60 jumps.

Principle #84

Incorporate weight-bearing exercises into your routine.

While all exercise is good, weight-bearing exercises, which force you to work against gravity, strengthen your bones more than others. Any exercise that is high impact will strengthen your bones. Brisk walking, running, stair-climbing, and weight-lifting all strengthen the skeletal system by putting weight on it. Aerobic exercises such as biking, rowing, or swimming are excellent for the cardiovascular system but do not strengthen your bones. Since some high-impact activities can put stress on other parts of your body (such as your knees), be sure to consult your doctor as you build your bone-strengthening exercise program.

Principle #85

Don't let soda rot your bones.

In addition to being loaded with calories and chemicals, soda is believed to rot your bones — literally. Researchers, such as bone expert Dr. James Duke, have found that phosphoric acid, found in most sodas, extracts calcium from bones, making them weaken prematurely. This puts people, especially women, at risk for various bone disorders, including osteoporosis, in addition to damaging arteries. Avoid this fate by eliminating soda from your diet.

Principle #86

Stretch to stay limber.

Beginning in our 30s, we lose flexibility. This is around the time when our muscles begin to tighten and shorten, giving us shorter range of motion. Maintaining flexibility allows us to do the exercises that help strengthen our bones and thus are part and parcel of maintaining a healthy skeletal system. To counteract loss of flexibility, incorporate yoga into your physical routine. Yoga works all the centers of the body and increases flexibility in just a few weeks. There are many simple poses you can do at home while watching television or before bed.

Principle #87

Eat a diet rich in vitamin D and calcuim.

Bones are strengthened by minerals that are cyclically lost and replaced over time. After 35, however, more minerals are lost than replaced, beginning the weakening of bones that continues through the rest of your life. To counteract the loss of bone minerals, increase your intake of bone nutrients. Calcium and vitamin D help preserve bone density and can be found in servings of milk, yogurt, almonds, and cheese. Or, take daily calcium and vitamin D supplements to ensure your bones get the nutrients they need.

Principle #88

Stop time by lifting weights.

Lifting weights is possibly the most important way to keep your bones and muscles strong as you age. In fact, one groundbreaking study out of the Center for Physical Activity and Nutrition at the School of Nutrition at Tufts University found that the bodies of 40 postmenopausal women became 15 to 20 years more youthful after they lifted weights twice a week for a year. Lifting weights doesn't mean you have to hang with bodybuilders at the gym. Try getting 1- to 2-pound ankle weights to wear while you walk, or do arm curls with 4- to 5-pound weights as you watch television.

Principle #89

Sit up straight.

One effect of bone density loss is poor posture. In fact, men begin losing height as early as their 40s. This is because fluid-filled disks that keep the spine elongated become dried out with age and collapse. By the time a man has reached the age of 60, he will have likely shrunk about 1.25 inches from his tallest height. You can improve the function of spinal disks by standing and sitting up straight. Also, learn to do yoga poses that elongate the spine — there are several. In addition to preventing shrinking, improving your posture will help you appear thinner.

Principle #90

Realize that smoking turns your bones to ash.

For years, smoking has been known to increase a woman's risk for developing osteoporosis. But new studies show that smoking also erodes the bones of men and that secondhand smoke increases the risk of developing osteoporosis in both genders. A 2006 study that measured bone density in more than 1,000 Swedish men aged 18 to 20 found that in smokers, bone density in the spine, hip, and overall body was as much as 5 percent lower than in nonsmokers their age. So consider improving your bone density among the many reasons to quit smoking today.

Principle #91

Get a bone density test.

Advances in technology have given doctors access to a bone density test that can determine a person's risk of osteoporosis while there is still time to improve bone strength. A bone density test uses special X-rays to measure how much bone mineral content is packed into a segment of bone — the higher the mineral content, the denser the bone. It is recommended that women over 65, or those at high risk for osteoporosis (those with family history, low body weight, a history of bone breakage, etc.), get bone density tests. Consult your doctor regarding whether a bone density test is right for you.

AVOIDING TOXINS

Recent statistics show that in the United States, 1 in 3 people have cancer, and 1 in 4 will die from it. In addition, 1 in 8 women will develop breast cancer, while 17 million people have asthma. Furthermore, 1 in 6 American children suffer from a developmental, learning, or behavioral disability, such as autism, Down's Syndrome, mental retardation, or Attention Deficit Disorder, and 4.6 million adults have Alzheimer's disease. No one knows exactly what causes each of these debilitating diseases, but more and more fingers are being pointed at the increasingly toxic environment in which we live.

Much of this toxicity comes from industrial pollution that has saturated our air, water, land, and food. As Americans, we are particularly at risk: more than 77,000 chemicals are produced in the U.S. and more than 1,000 new ones are introduced each year. Where do all of these chemicals go? Because many of them are used in the food industry (as pesticides, herbicides, fungicides, or for food processing), they are absorbed into groundwater, rivers, lakes, bays, swamps, and oceans. They are also absorbed into the soil or buried in the earth. Factories spew toxic chemicals into the air, and many — more than 10,000 toxic chemicals — are added to foods we eat to process or preserve them.

Many of these toxins are in forms we cannot see, taste, or smell, which adds to their deadly effect. We don't realize we have been hurt by long-term exposure to toxins until we come down with a chronic, life-threatening disease. Start learning today about what toxins you are exposed to on a daily basis. Discover what toxins may be in your environment. What goes into the food you eat? What chemicals are in the lotion you put on your skin? How might bottled water introduce more toxins into your body? The following principles provide information on these and other sources of toxins and help you begin today to avoid them for a healthier and longer life.

PRINCIPLE #92

Skip the trans fats.

Trans fats are acids found in hydrogenated and partially hydrogenated oils, which are used to improve taste and prolong the shelf-life of a food product. These oils have been used in place of butter and coconut oils because they are cheaper to process. But the trans fat acids contained in these oils are toxic and increase the risk of heart disease, cancer, diabetes, obesity, infertility, and even death. Trans fats are commonly found in cake mixes, microwave popcorn, peanut butter, frozen pizza, taco shells, and hundreds of other processed products. To be sure you avoid them, carefully read labels — if the word "hydrogenated" appears anywhere, skip that food.

PRINCIPLE #93

Limit your consumption of fish exposed to pollution.

Fish is recommended by the American Heart Association as an important source of omega-3 fatty acids, which are good for the heart. But some fish may contain high levels of mercury, PCBs (polychlorinated biphenyls), dioxins, and other contaminants from water pollution. Ingesting high levels of mercury and PCBs may cause birth defects and cancer. Levels of these substances tend to be highest in older, larger fish, and the highest levels of mercury are found in shark, swordfish, tuna, mackerel, and red snapper. Above all, avoid farm-raised salmon, which are fed meals of ground-up fish with high PCB contamination.

Principle #94

Switch to natural body products and cosmetics.

We often forget that our skin is the largest organ of the body. It's not just a pretty exterior — our skin functions as a giant sponge that absorbs whatever is put on it. Many lotions, shampoos, hair dyes, cosmetics, and other beauty products are loaded with carcinogens and irritants that get absorbed into the body through the skin. These carcinogens include lead, formaldehyde, and coal tar, which have been found to cause health problems such as headaches, asthma, and cancer. To prevent your skin from absorbing harmful toxins, switch to a line of natural or organic body care products — many are available online or in your local health store.

Principle #95

Beware of mold.

If you live by a body of water (as do more than 110 million Americans), chances are your humid environment facilitates the growth of mold. Many molds contain mycotoxins, which can cause a wide range of health problems, including cancer, heart disease, asthma, multiple sclerosis, diabetes, and even death. If you have a mold problem anywhere in your home, get it tested by a professional. He or she will be able to tell you the source of the mold, how dangerous it is, and how to prevent it from coming back.

Principle #96

Bottled is not always better.

Bottled water is a convenient way to stay hydrated on the go. But most people are unaware that plastic water bottles are made with chemicals called phthalates, which leak in microscopic amounts. Phthalates damage the endocrine system and may contribute to certain cancers. Instead of bottled water, install a water-cleansing filter onto your tap; these effectively remove chemicals and minerals from tap water without leaking them into your supply. Or, sign up for water service delivery, or buy a refrigerator with a built-in water filter. For water on the go, buy a polyurethane bottle, often found at outdoors stores. These do not leak phthalates and are dishwasher safe.

PRINCIPLE #97

Buy organic produce.

A 2002 study published in the journal Food Additives and Contaminants showed that eating organic produce exposes a person to ⅓ as many pesticide residues than commercially grown foods. Though organic produce is more expensive, eating it is an excellent way to prevent cancer, nerve damage, birth defects, and other negative effects of pesticides. If your budget doesn't allow you to buy everything organic, start with items that have an edible peel, such as red peppers and apples. Bananas and oranges are less important to buy organic because the fruit is protected by their thick peel.

Principle #98

Use natural cleaning products in your home.

Many cleaning products, disinfectants, varnishes, and paints contain dangerous compounds called volatile organic compounds (VOC). VOCs are emitted as gases from solids or liquids. According to the Environmental Protection Agency, when released indoors their concentration is dangerously high (10 times higher than outdoors) and can contribute to cancer; liver, kidney, and central nervous system damage; as well as eye irritation, respiratory ailments, headaches, dizziness, visual problems, and memory impairment. So replace your fleet of cleaning products and fresheners with a line of products that is natural or organic, found online or in most health stores.

PRINCIPLE #99

Fast periodically.

Centuries ago, ancient Qigong Taoists identified what they called the "toxins of 3 dead bodies." These are toxins they believed were present in the dead bodies of animals, plants, and microbes. Because they couldn't avoid eating anything without toxins, Qigong Taoists routinely fasted to cleanse their bodies. You don't have to be a Taoist to fast — religious and medical practitioners agree that occasional fasting can clear the body of accumulated toxins. Fasts can last 1 day or 1 week. Some involve a detoxifying drink of lemon juice and cayenne pepper, others allow raw foods to be consumed. Consult your doctor to find a fast that's right for you.

Principle #100

Love your liver.

———————— ✳ ————————

The liver has been called the workhorse of the human body; it performs more than 500 functions, the most important of which is processing nutrients and toxins from your body. Indeed, everything you consume is processed through your liver. Should your liver become damaged, however, it will not process toxins as efficiently, and they will back up in your body, causing diabetes, blood disease, and hypoglycemia. So take care of your workhorse! Avoid alcohol, caffeine, pesticides, food colorings, and fatty meats, as they all hurt the liver's ability to function properly. Foods that help detoxify the liver include beets, lemons, broccoli, eggs, walnuts, and caraway seeds.

PRINCIPLE #101

Use fiber to show toxins the door.

※

Eating fiber is another way to cleanse your body of toxins. Fiber is the part of food your body can't digest. Fiber is like the train on which toxins catch a ride out of your body; toxins and useless nutrients bond to fiber, which is then passed through your biological systems. Eating a diet high in fiber will help you eliminate the toxins from your body and reduce your risk of cardiovascular disease. Foods high in fiber include whole-wheat breads, wheat cereals, wheat bran, rye, rice, barley, cabbage, beets, carrots, turnips, cauliflower, and apples.

REDUCING STRESS

According to the Centers for Disease Control, the leading 6 causes of death in the U.S. — heart disease, cancer, lung ailments, accidents, cirrhosis of the liver, and suicide — are all brought on at least in part by stress. To avoid these and other debilitating diseases, it is critical that you get your stress levels under control.

Reducing stress is not that easy in a 24/7 society like ours. Studies show that Americans are some of the most stressed out people on the entire planet. Why? Data from the United Nations indicates that Americans work some of the longest hours of workers in all industrialized countries. Work hours are up, while vacation hours are down; American employers offer some of the poorest vacation plans in the industrialized world. Every other country with an economy comparable to the United States' guarantees paid vacation to its workforce. Britain allows its workforce 20 days of guaranteed, paid leave. Germany offers 24 days of paid vacation, and France gives 30 days. Employers in the U.S. typically offer about 12, and they are not obligated to guarantee any paid leave at all. Even those who are offered more vacation do not necessarily take it; each year, there is a segment of the population that forfeits their annual vacation allowance because they don't have the time or money to take a break.

Furthermore, Americans have embraced the high-tech, plugged-in gadgets of our time that keep them on the go. Our demanding schedules naturally lead to us to experience high levels of stress, which is detrimental to both our physical and emotional health.

In addition to shortening your life span and putting you at increased risk for disease, experiencing chronic stress reduces your quality of life. Stressed people report being more angry, tired, and depressed than non-stressed people. Therefore, learning how to practice relaxation and stress management is integral to increasing your levels of peace, happiness, and energy. To feel better and enjoy your day-to-day life, you must get your stress under control. Use the following simple principles to start doing so today.

PRINCIPLE #102

Quiet your mind.

Take a few minutes to consider how noise contributes to your stress level. Even in our homes, we are constantly barraged by the sounds of nearby construction, landscaping, car alarms, planes, sirens, and household noises such as televisions, kitchen instruments, and laundry machines. According to the Citizens Coalition Against Noise Pollution, "Daily levels of noise pollution cause hearing loss, stress, hypertension, increased blood pressure and headaches. High-frequency noise can cause permanent hearing damage; low-frequency noise produces pressure waves that can cause nausea and heart palpitations." Make time for quiet every day to give yourself a chance to de-stress and reset.

Principle #103

Surround yourself with stress-free images.

—— ❋ ——

Your mind processes millions of images every day. These images are like data fed into a computer. Your brain is the computer — be sure to upload it with images that relax and de-stress you. Make your home visually relaxing. Decorate using cool, relaxing colors such as blues, purples, and greens (avoid reds and oranges, which stimulate the appetite). Hang pictures of whatever relaxes you — images of family and friends or vistas of natural beauty. Keep items that heighten your stress levels — such as bills, work, or medical items — in a separate corner of the house that you visit infrequently.

Principle #104

Express anger before it turns to rage.

Anger, frustration, and rage are key sources of stress. Everyone feels angry sometimes, but you can greatly reduce stress by expressing your anger before it festers. A Buddhist proverb states, "Holding on to anger is like grasping a hot coal with the intent of throwing it at someone else; you are the one who gets burned." Indeed, holding onto anger and collecting things to be angry about quickly leads to high levels of stress, which jeopardize your quality of life. Therefore, deal with small annoyances as they come rather than waiting until you explode with rage.

PRINCIPLE #105

Just breathe.

When you feel stress coming on, take deep breaths that start low in your belly. Exhale until every drop of breath has left your lungs. This type of deep, rhythmic breathing expands the diaphragm muscle, the cone-shaped muscle below your lungs that aids in respiration. The lung's air pockets become filled, and this allows you to take in more oxygen and release more carbon dioxide with each breath. The end result is more oxygen flows to your brain and lymphatic systems, which releases endorphins, the body's natural pain killers and relaxants. When you are stressed, deep breathing will ease you into a state of physical calm; your mood will surely follow.

Principle #106

Keep your home and office organized.

— ❄ —

Being organized reduces the stress that comes from not knowing where to find something in a pinch. Clutter not only takes up physical space, but it also negatively affects your mental health. So put the dishes away after you wash them. Fold and put away laundry. Hang your coat up when you take it off. Clear off your desk at the end of the day. Have a pen and paper handy near the phone. When you're finished with something, put it back where it belongs. Keeping your surroundings in order will help you live a stress-free life.

Principle #107

Unplug yourself.

※

Stress is a widespread problem in our world where everyone is constantly "plugged in." People spend their waking hours tied to email, BlackBerries, cell phones, computers, and other instruments that keep them on the go. If this is your lifestyle, be sure to spend time every day unplugged. For just 20 minutes, turn your phone off, shut your laptop, and spend the time taking a quick nap or a relaxing walk. In addition to feeling better, your employer will thank you: According to the Centers for Disease Control, U.S. employers spend $300 billion ($7,500 per employee) each year on stress-related issues, including reduced productivity, absenteeism, health insurance costs, and employee turnover.

Principle #108

Treat yourself to a massage.

— ✳ —

Few activities alleviate stress like getting a massage. Massage therapy helps to relieve tension headaches, eyestrain, muscle tension, and stiffness. Massage is so effective one recent poll found that 54 percent of primary care physicians and family practitioners said they would encourage their patients to pursue massage therapy as a complement to medical treatments. And, massages do not have to be expensive. Many massage schools offer discounted services so their students can practice their skills. An additional idea is to ask a friend or partner to exchange massages. If you do not find massages appealing, try indulging in another relaxing activity to reduce stress, such as a daytime nap or a long, hot bath.

Principle #109

Cultivate your hobbies.

— ✳ —

Make time each week for a hobby that you find relaxing. For instance, take a painting class or learn how to build model trains — you will likely find it satisfying to work with your hands and produce something beautiful. Hobbies have been medically proven to reduce stress. One study of 30 female heart patients discussed in the *American Journal Medical Association* showed a significant decrease in heart rate, blood pressure, and perspiration rate while the subjects worked on a simple craft project. So take time out to pursue a hobby you enjoy — it will make you feel better and lengthen your life span.

PRINCIPLE #110

Stick to your budget.

According to the American Psychological Association, 73 percent of Americans list money as the number one factor that affects their stress level. Therefore, it is good practice to live within your means. Establish a budget and stick to it. If you cannot afford to purchase something nonessential with cash, don't buy it. Put items on your credit cards only when you know you can pay off the whole balance when you receive the bill. Sticking to a budget means you may not have a fancy new outfit or new DVD, but you will achieve the peace of mind that comes with not being in debt.

Principle #111

Ditch the workaholic life.

Writer Margaret Fuller once noted, "Men for the sake of getting a living forget to live." If you find yourself devoting inordinate chunks of time to work, ask yourself, what are you getting out of it? Refrain from working more than 9 hours a day and take at least 1 day a week to do no work at all. Instead of working yourself to the bone, make sure the hours you spend at work are of quality. The world is not likely to fall apart if you do not check your email or return a phone call immediately, so there is no sense to add such stress to your life.

KEEPING YOUR MIND SHARP

Imagine your brain as a big, damp sponge that is squeezed as you age. When the sponge becomes older it gets exposed to substances that remove moisture from it. When the sponge becomes dried out, pieces break off and it becomes smaller. This is much like what happens to the aging brain if it is not cared for. Thus, it is your responsibility to keep your brain from "drying out" in order to feel better and live a longer life.

Loss of brain mass is common among the elderly and causes unhappiness, sickness, and premature death. As their brain loses mass, older adults find they have difficulty remembering and concentrating. Damage to brain mass also results in what researchers call "sensory integration dysfunction." Sensory integration dysfunction is when your brain combines information from all of your senses at once, making it difficult to focus on a specific task. For instance, when in a restaurant, an older person may have trouble simultaneously eating his dinner and hearing the conversation going on at his table. This is because he unable to tease out the discussion from all of the other conversations going on in the room. In addition, the many sights and smells present in the room become overwhelming and distracting. As his senses become overloaded, he may forget to eat or seem out of sorts.

This fate does not have to become yours, however. There are many things you can do now to strengthen your brain so that it stays strong and capable as you age. A great way to ward off cognitive decline is to practice keeping your mind sharp by doing word puzzles as well as by playing games, reading, eating a healthy diet, and exercising. People should also limit their time in front of televisions and computers. A study conducted by Dr. Amir Soas of Case Western Reserve University Medical School suggests, "Start a new hobby or learn to speak a foreign language. Anything that stimulates the brain to think. Also, watch less television, because your brain goes into neutral." In another study, 6-year-old children who were given music lessons scored higher on IQ tests compared with kids who did not receive music lessons — this was because learning music helped sharpen their minds. Yet another study found that preschool-age children had higher spatial reasoning scores after 2 years of music lessons than children who were given computer lessons.

There is no way to stop the aging process, but there are definite steps you can take now to protect your brain from debilitating diseases such as Alzheimer's and dementia. Use the following simple principles as a jumping-off point to get started keeping your mind sharp as you age.

PRINCIPLE #112

Fine-tune your memory.

An excellent way to combat memory loss is to learn a musical instrument. A study in the international research journal *Medical Science Monitor* found that "active participation in a group keyboard program was far more effective at reversing stress signatures [which cause memory loss] than simply relaxing and reading newspapers and magazines." The skill of reading music, too, has been proven to keep the mind alert and focused. In addition, learning to play an instrument is an engaging and pleasant endeavor. You are sure to find yourself feeling satisfied as you master both your instrument and your mind.

Principle #113

Do concentration calisthenics.

Word games like Scrabble and Boggle can dust off mental cobwebs by keeping your mind alert and functioning. Such games force you to practice the twin skills of concentration and resisting distraction. The jumble of letters causes you to concoct combinations and improve your vocabulary, which keeps your brain active. Puzzles such as crosswords and Sudoku are also great for practicing your concentration skills. *AARP Magazine* also recommends jigsaw puzzles for improving "spatial intelligence," a high-level problem-solving skill. Even if you only put a few pieces together each day, your brain is getting a workout.

Principle #114

Dump the doldrums by switching jobs.

Nothing will kill concentration, creativity, and a genuine will to stay sharp like a dead-end job. A dead-end job is one in which you are neither challenged nor engaged. Studies show a droning day-to-day existence contributes to depression, which in turn causes difficulty concentrating, remembering, and making decisions. Over time, this state of feeling will inevitably result in a dull mind. If you find yourself staring down a dead-end job, make a change. Many people start to experience immediate brain stimulation when they simply look at job ads.

PRINCIPLE #115

Learn a foreign language.

The cognitive benefits of learning a foreign language are extensive. Studies show that children enrolled in foreign language programs do better in school and are more creative than those who are not. Several studies also show that people who know more than 1 language score higher on IQ tests. One study conducted by London's Wellcome Department of Imaging Neuroscience found that brain imaging showed bilingual speakers had denser gray matter compared with those who spoke just 1 language — and gray matter density indicates better language, memory, and attention skills. So whether it is *français*, *español*, *deutsch*, or *italiano*, start learning a foreign language today.

PRINCIPLE #116

Charge your batteries by changing your routine.

We've all resorted to "autopilot" while driving to work. In fact, many of us could get ourselves to work blindfolded. Engaging in the same activities in the same way every day causes your brain to become lazy. So, the next time you drive to work, take a different route. Making small changes to your daily routine will ignite little-used brain connectors and get them fired up and running again. Other ways to avoid routine behavior include rearranging the furniture in your house, switching closets with your partner, parking in a different spot than your usual space, and changing the order of your morning routine.

Principle #117

Eat smart foods.

Many of us do not realize that when we sit down to a meal, we feed our brain along with the rest of our body. The human brain uses up to 20 percent of the total calories that you take in each day. Therefore, it is important to eat foods that will literally feed your mind. Mounting evidence suggests that omega-3 fatty acids and docosahexaenoic acid (DHA) improve brain functioning and stave off dementia. These are found in eggs and fish. Other "brain foods" include broccoli, strawberries, and blueberries. In one study, rats fed a steady diet of strawberries and blueberries demonstrated improved coordination, concentration, and short-term memory over those who were not.

PRINCIPLE #118

Clear your head.

Going for a walk to clear your head is not just an expression. In fact, walking is a great and easy way to nourish your mind. Walking increases blood circulation, which brings oxygen to your brain. Increased circulation also carries glucose to your brain, which provides the energy it needs to function. Since walking is not strenuous, the extra oxygen and glucose are not sucked up by your muscles as they would be during more taxing forms of exercise. Tellingly, a University of California, San Francisco study found a dramatic halt to cognitive decline among elderly women who walked at least a half-mile each week.

Principle #119

Switch hands and close your eyes.

Researchers at The Franklin Institute have discovered that forcing yourself to switch hands or to engage in everyday activities with your eyes closed can help stimulate neuron growth. Neurons are cells that send and receive electrochemical signals to and from the brain and nervous system. To stimulate neuron growth, engage in activities such as using your nondominant hand to maneuver the computer mouse, to eat, or to brush your hair and teeth. Get dressed with your eyes closed, using only your hands to figure out buttons and zippers. Enjoy your meal in silence with your eyes closed, and savor each flavor.

Principle #120

Remember out loud.

Perhaps the most fun way to exercise your brain is to tell stories. Storytelling is an ancient art that has evolved over the centuries. You can continue it by developing your own style. Becoming a great storyteller helps keep your mind sharp by forcing you to recall details that add flavor to a tale. Furthermore, it stimulates imagination — both yours and your audience's. Additionally, researchers have found that explaining concepts to others solidifies them in the minds of both the listener and the speaker. Think of sharing your life's stories with others as backing up your memory hard drive.

Preventing Illness

It is often said that an ounce of prevention is worth a pound of cure. In other words, doing a little bit in advance to prevent something bad from happening can save you time, effort, money, and heartache later on down the road. This is the perspective you must adopt regarding your health if you seek to live a happier, healthier, and longer life.

Preventing illness means taking care of your body throughout your life and being proactive about visiting health care professionals to detect problems early on. Indeed, early detection of some diseases, such as cancer, is the key determinant in whether a person will live, suffer, or die. Consider that detecting oral cancer early can improve a person's chance of surviving it from 50 percent to more than 80 percent. Likewise, 85 percent of cervical cancer cases can be successfully treated when caught early; prostate cancer has a nearly 100 percent survival rate when detected early. Doctors estimate that if all Americans over

50 submitted to a colonoscopy once every decade, early detection could prevent 90 percent of the annual 150,000 colorectal cancer diagnoses and 50,000 deaths from the disease. Clearly, being proactive with cancer-detecting diagnostic tests and exams can mean the difference between life and death.

Yet many Americans choose not to take steps to prevent illness. Men especially dislike going to the doctor; surveys show they avoid doctor visits because it makes them feel powerless, less manly, and out of control. And Americans of both genders hate visiting the dentist even more; according to the Dental Phobia Treatment Center, 50 percent of the American public does not seek regular dental care. An estimated 9 to 15 percent of all Americans avoid the dentist altogether due to anxiety and fear of the visit. This means between 30 and 40 million people do not visit the dentist because they are afraid.

Fearing doctors and dentists is all the more reason to visit them more frequently — so you can stay out of their offices later in life. Use the following simple principles to proactively prevent illness so you can feel happier, healthier, and live longer.

PRINCIPLE #121

Wash your hands at every opportunity.

— ❋ —

Viruses and bacteria collect on our hands and make us sick when we touch our face. Just some of the situations in which to wash your hands include preparing or eating food, using the bathroom, cleaning, blowing your nose, coughing, sneezing, or handling waste. Interestingly, an American Society for Microbiology study found that people do not wash their hands as often as they should. While 91 percent of adults claim to wash their hands after using the restroom, only 82 percent actually do. Also, 90 percent of women wash their hands regularly, but just 75 percent of men do. Keeping hands clean prevents illness.

PRINCIPLE #122

Get diagnostic tests.

Everyone knows to go for annual checkups at the doctor. But equally important is to follow through with diagnostic tests that can catch diseases such as cancer early on. For women, it is important to get annual Pap smears after the age of 18, practice monthly breast exams, and get mammograms annually at age 40 (or if you know you are at high risk for breast cancer, at age 35). Men should get colonoscopies annually beginning at age 40, or at age 35 if there is high risk. Everyone should have EKGs when recommended by physicians. Diagnostic tests help catch cancer early on and can truly make the difference between life and death.

Principle #123

Know your restaurants.

———————— ❉ ————————

Each year, thousands are sickened by food-borne illnesses from eating in unsanitary restaurants. States that lead the nation in outbreaks of restaurant-related food poisonings are Florida, California, Ohio, Michigan, New York, and Minnesota, according to Healthinspections.com. Some illnesses are caused by eating produce or meat tainted with E. coli, Norovirus, or salmonella. Other illnesses spring from unsanitary kitchen conditions or from employees failing to wash equipment or their hands. Food-borne illnesses range from a common cold to severe diarrhea, dehydration, and even death. Make sure you can trust the restaurants you go to by checking their inspection rating (many states require scores to be visibly posted) or reading reviews.

Principle #124

Use supplements to supplement, not replace.

Taking supplements such as echinacea and vitamin C are believed to strengthen your immune system by helping you resist colds and flus. Furthermore, taking a multivitamin can help you get the vitamins and minerals you need on a daily basis, regardless of how you eat. However, supplements should live up to their name — they should supplement a healthy diet, not serve as a replacement for one. In fact, a study from the Harvard School of Public Health showed that although taking higher doses of vitamin B6, vitamin B12, and vitamin D have health benefits, taking supplements cannot erase the health effects of a poor diet and a sedentary lifestyle.

Principle #125

Don't inhale an early death.

———————————— ✳ ————————————

Smoking is, hands down, the worst activity you can engage in. Smoking contributes to the development of almost all diseases, including cancer, emphysema, heart disease, high blood pressure, high cholesterol, diabetes, and asthma. It also lowers immunity, making you more likely to get sick; puts limits on your physical abilities; causes snoring and sleep apnea; and impairs fine motor skills, to name a few effects. The good news is that quitting smoking before any of the above diseases become chronic can, with time, reverse the ill effects on your health.

PRINCIPLE #126

Sweat out sickness.

While smoking is probably the worst thing you can do for your body, exercise is no doubt the best. Exercising regularly prevents a long list of diseases, including cancer, heart disease, stroke, high blood pressure, vascular disease, diabetes, obesity, and osteoporosis. Exercise also prevents mental health disorders, including depression, anxiety, and stress. Finally, exercising strengthens your immune system, providing defense against common colds and influenza. To prevent illness, feel better, and live longer, make exercise your lifelong friend.

Principle #127

Practice oral care.

———————— ❋ ————————

Brushing and flossing regularly prevent cavities and periodontitis (gum disease). Avoiding such ills not only gives you a whiter, brighter smile but also clean, inviting breath. If left untreated, periodontitis can erode the gum, jaw bone, and supporting tissue around teeth. Furthermore, periodontal-disease bacteria can enter your bloodstream and travel through your body, causing troubles such as heart disease, diabetes, and respiratory disease. As Spanish author Miguel de Cervantes once said, "Every tooth in a man's head is more valuable than a diamond." Be sure to treat yours well.

Principle #128

Establish your personal physical baseline.

An excellent way to prevent illness is to become acutely aware of how your body reacts in times of sickness and health. Do this by keeping a wellness journal. When you are healthy, write down how you feel. What is your body temperature? How much energy do you have? What is your appetite? What level of pain, if any, do you feel? Likewise, when ill, take note of your condition and symptoms. By establishing your personal physical baseline you will be able to tell when illness is coming on and thus react quickly. Knowing your body will also allow you to better communicate your symptoms to your physician.

PRINCIPLE #129

Maintain a clean environment.

Cleaning the house is not just so it looks nice for company, it is to prevent you and your family from getting sick! Regularly dusting, vacuuming, mopping, and polishing can prevent the growth of mold, bacteria, and dust mites. The presence of these contributes to asthma, allergies, and other illnesses that remove our ability to feel our best. So make cleaning a part of your daily regimen. Also, if there are pets in the house, make sure they are bathed regularly and receive topical or oral flea and parasite control.

PRINCIPLE #130

Know your family history.

Many diseases are hereditary, or passed genetically through generations. It is important to learn what diseases you are at risk of developing by knowing your family history. Knowing your family's history of disease can help your physician diagnose problems early; it can also help you change your lifestyle to minimize your risk. For example, if you know you are prone to high cholesterol, make dietary changes early in life. If you know breast cancer runs in your family, get mammograms earlier than the recommended age of 40. Ask your parents and grandparents what diseases run in your family so you are prepared to face them head on.

THE BENEFITS OF
SEX AND TOUCH

When the conversation turns to sex, many Americans find themselves embarrassed, shy, or even offended. As author Don Schrader once wrote, "To hear many religious people talk, one would think God created the torso, head, legs and arms, but the devil slapped on the genitals." But understanding the benefits regular and safe sex can have on your life is one of the most important things you can do to feel better and even live longer.

Indeed, dozens of studies from some of the world's most reputable institutions have concluded that having sex with someone you care about can improve all areas of your life. It can help you lose weight, look prettier, smile brighter, and stand taller. Its benefits include a reduced risk of cancer, disease, heart attack, and stroke. Having sex gives you confidence, relaxes you, clears your mind, improves your ability to focus, and even reduces depression. Alexander

person who sought to publicize the advantages of a healthy sex life when he wrote *The Joy of Sex*, which helped herald the sexual revolution of the mid-20th century. Comfort hoped that because of its many benefits, humanity would "eventually come to realize that chastity is no more a virtue than malnutrition."

It is important to note that the benefits of sex are entirely contingent upon doing it safely, which means within the confines of a monogamous, loving relationship in which contraception and protection are used. In other words, for many of the following health benefits to take effect, you must practice safe sex. For men, safe sex has the ability to lower the risk of developing prostate cancer by as much as one-third. But having unsafe sex — such as sex without protection with someone whose sexual history is unfamiliar to you — actually increases a man's likelihood of developing cancer by as much as 40 percent, due to increased exposure to sexually transmitted diseases that can contribute to cancer. With this in mind, use the following principles safely and responsibly to maximize your ability to benefit from sex.

Principle #131

Use sex to take your mind off your problems.

It is no secret that intercourse relaxes both men and women. But having sex with your partner regularly can actually take your mind off your problems for hours. A hormone called oxytocin, which has an amnesic effect that lasts as long as 5 hours, triggers orgasms. So after sex, you are likely to be less troubled by work, bills, or other everyday stressors. Furthermore, when you go to solve these problems after sex, you are likely to approach them in a more relaxed, calm, and productive state.

PRINCIPLE #132

Shed pounds the fun way.

A tumble in the sack with your partner can burn up to 200 calories, the equivalent of putting in 15 minutes on a Stairmaster or going cross-country skiing. In fact, the pulse of an aroused person is about 150 beats per minute, the same as an athlete performing at top speed. Sex also works to tone the body: intercourse involves a series of intense muscular contractions that work the pelvis, thighs, buttocks, stomach, arms, neck, and thorax. Dr. Claire Bailey of the University of Bristol has said that regular sex can also improve a woman's posture. Finally, sex increases production of testosterone in men, which helps build stronger bones and muscles.

PRINCIPLE #133

Improve the quality of your relationship.

Many couples tend to refrain from having sex when they are not getting along. But studies show it is even more important to be intimate during troubled times. Each time you have a positive sexual experience with your partner, your brain associates him or her with pleasure. Your relationship can be improved simply by making time for intimacy together. As actress Mae West once quipped, "Sex is emotion in motion." Show your partner how much you care for him or her by engaging in intimacy often.

PRINCIPLE #134

Fight depression the natural way.

Multiple studies at reputable institutions have found that semen contains a hormone called prostaglandin that helps reduce depression in women. In fact, a 2002 State University of New York, Albany study on nearly 300 women found that those who had sex without condoms were less subject to depression than couples that did. Researchers explained the difference by arguing that prostaglandin was absorbed by the woman's genital tract. Once absorbed by the body, it stimulated female hormones that elevate mood. So fight off depression the natural way — become intimate with your partner tonight!

PRINCIPLE #135

Ward off cancer by having sex.

Studies show the more often men ejaculate, the lower their risk of prostate cancer. One study in the *British Journal of Urology International* found that men in their 20s reduce their chance of developing prostate cancer by 33 percent by ejaculating 5 or more times a week. This is because to make semen, male organs take minerals and carcinogens from the blood and concentrate them up to 600 times. They are then expunged from the body rather than lingering in the prostate. It is important to note that a man's risk of cancer increases by 40 percent if he practices unsafe sex, due to the possibility of contracting STDs. So only have safe or solo sex to ward off prostate cancer.

Principle #136

Use pleasure to live a pain-free life.

When both men and women orgasm, they release large amounts of natural chemicals such as endorphins, estrogen, and oxytocin, which dull pain. The pain-relieving properties of these chemicals in the bloodstream alleviate headaches and arthritis in men and women and pre-menstrual syndrome in women. In addition, women can increase the amount of pain they are able to tolerate by having regular orgasms. According to a study by professor Beverly Whipple of Rutgers University, women who masturbate to orgasm increase their pain tolerance threshold by 74.6 percent and their pain detection threshold by 106.7 percent.

PRINCIPLE #137

Love your way to a healthier heart.

Sex has been proven to boost cardiovascular health in both men and women. A 2001 Queens University study found that by having sex more than 3 times a week, men can reduce their risk of heart attack or stroke by 50 percent. The study also found that women who have more sex produce higher levels of estrogen, which protects against heart disease. Furthermore, women who indulged their partners in oral sex have been found to be at lower risk for developing preeclampsia, a dangerously high blood pressure syndrome that can accompany pregnancy.

Principle #138

Love every day keeps the doctor away.

Nothing makes us feel worse than being slammed with sickness. The good news is that having sex can help ward off common illnesses, helping you feel better in several ways. Researchers at Wilkes University in Pennsylvania say individuals who have sex at least a couple times a week have 30 percent higher levels of an antibody called immunoglobulin A, which boosts the immune system. Sex is also reported to be a natural antihistamine, helping combat hay fever, asthma, and congestion. So make sure to include time for intimacy in your life — sex, plus an apple, is sure to keep the doctor away.

Principle #139

Look better, feel better, love better.

※

Most of us focus our attention on looking good before we have sex. But studies show that frequent sex helps improve our appearance in many ways. When women orgasm they produce extra levels of the hormone estrogen. Increased estrogen makes hair shiny and soft (and also helps prevent osteoporosis and Alzheimer's disease). Furthermore, increased levels of serotonin give the skin a rosy, healthy glow. Finally, sex can even whiten your smile: Minerals contained in semen — zinc, calcium, and others — have been shown in several authoritative studies to slow tooth decay in women who indulge their partners in oral sex.

PRINCIPLE #140

Live longer with your loved one.

Possibly the most impressive benefit of sex with a loved one is that it can increase your life span. One study at Queens University in Belfast, Ireland, tracked the health of 1,000 middle-aged men for 10 years. It concluded that men who reported having orgasms most often had a death rate of 50 percent less than those who did not. Of these results, co-author of the study, Dr. Shah Ebrahim, said, "The relationship found between frequency of sexual intercourse and mortality is of considerable public interest." So make time to make love with your partner — it will help you enjoy each other's company for additional years to come.

Principle #141

Don't be afraid to masturbate.

It is important to note that masturbation, or solo sex, can achieve most, if not all, of the benefits that sex offers. Achieving orgasm by yourself can elevate your mood, relax and calm you, help tone muscles, prevent cancer, result in pain relief, help your heart, improve your skin and hair, boost your immune system, and even add years to your life. More important, practicing solo sex helps you get comfortable with your body, which is helpful for when you become intimate with another person. So don't be afraid to use masturbation to feel better.

Getting in Touch with Your Spiritual Side

In their quest for a healthier, happier, and longer life, many people overlook the importance of spirituality. Do not make this mistake: getting in touch with your spiritual side is one of the most profound ways in which you can improve the way you feel in both the short and long term. In fact, not only does a sense of spirituality help reduce the stress, tension, and fear that make us feel worse every day, but it will help you outlive those who do not share your sense of spirituality.

Studies have repeatedly shown the connection between faith, spirituality, and longer life. One study reported in the *New York Times* showed that people with faith who suffer from life-threatening ailments recover faster and live longer than those who do not. Said the *Times*: "In a study of 232 elderly patients who had undergone open-heart surgery, those who were able to find strength and comfort in their religious outlook had a survival rate 3 times higher than those who found no balm in religious faith."

Developing a sense of spirituality can also help establish and guide your values, which in turn allows you to feel great about the life you live. From spirituality and religion, people derive a sense of right and wrong. They cultivate a set of standards to live up to, such as being a good, generous, decent person. They are more likely to treat family, friends, and even strangers with respect. Through religious and spiritual practices, they develop a sense of responsibility and respect for history, fellow humans, and the environment. Each of these beliefs works to inform your understanding of the world and your role in it, which allows you to feel purposeful and happy.

Getting in touch with your spiritual side is a lifelong pursuit that will take time, introspection, and energy. Use the following principles to steer you in the direction of developing a sense of spirituality that will help you feel better and live longer.

Principle #142

Realize that a sense of spirituality can help you live longer.

According to a study commissioned by the National Institutes of Health, those who regularly attend church or another house of worship have a significantly reduced mortality rate than people who do not. In other words, having spirituality helps you live longer! Scientists are trying to pinpoint why this is so. Some believe the extended life span is due to the strong social community and healthy lifestyle churchgoers tend to enjoy. No matter the reason, take comfort in the fact that your spirituality is helping you enjoy your days on earth and give you more of them.

Principle #143

Learn to see evidence of
the divine all around you.

An old proverb states, "Faith is like electricity — we cannot see it, but we can see the light." Indeed, those who deny the existence of a divine spirit are bound to miss the evidence of one, but if you are spiritually in tune with your community, you will see the proof all around you. On some days this might be a beautiful sunset; on others it might be a connection with a long-lost friend. There are millions of ways to see evidence of the divine every day — but you must be looking for it.

PRINCIPLE #144

Don't worry if you struggle with your faith.

If you struggle with your faith, you are not alone. In one study of spiritual people, more than 80 percent admitted to, at some point, doubting that God exists. But part of being human is experiencing periods of doubt and confusion. If your faith falters now and then, remind yourself that while no one can prove there is a god, no one can prove there isn't. As the Reverend Robert Schuller once put it, "I would rather err on the side of faith than on the side of doubt." So err on the side of faith for a more meaningful existence.

PRINCIPLE #145

Believe in a grand plan.

✳

The philosopher Rabindranath Tagore once said, "Faith is the bird that feels the light when the dawn is still dark." Indeed, putting your trust in the existence of what you cannot see is difficult at times, but important. Believing in a grand plan helps humans understand the chaos of life, including death, tragedy, and inequality. Finding meaning through believing in a grand plan will help alleviate spiritual crises and bring joy, meaning, and purpose to your life.

Principle #146

Respect the Ten Commandments, and add to them.

———————— ✳ ————————

Even if you do not belong to any particular religion, the basic ethical principles summarized in the Ten Commandments are good rules by which to live a righteous and meaningful life. This is why all the world's major theologies incorporate these basic tenants in some way. Everyone can agree that it is right to honor your family and community and to refrain from lying, cheating, stealing, adultery, and murder. Feel free to tailor the idea of commandments by adding principles that are especially important to you, such as, "I will be kind to animals," or "I will respect the environment."

PRINCIPLE #147

Realize that having faith makes you intelligent.

❈

Many people struggle with the part of faith that requires them to accept ideas that cannot be proven. But never let anyone tell you that having faith is a mark of unintelligence. In fact, according to Planet Project, a polling company that surveyed 380,000 people in more than 225 countries, highly educated people are more likely to believe in God. Of those polled, 63 percent of those who said they believe in God had a secondary-school education, while 72 percent of believers held a college degree.

Principle #148

Turn to your spirituality to get you through the dark times.

An old proverb states, "Fear knocked at the door. Faith answered. And no one was there." Indeed, there is no more important time to have spirituality than when you are filled with fear, doubt, and sorrow. Your faith can help you conquer each of these demons. So look to the sky when all you can see is the ground. Turn your head up and believe that you are not alone. It is during your most difficult times that you need your faith, so keep your head up and feel God's comforting presence.

Principle #149

Look beyond organized religion for spirituality.

Many Americans have rejected organized religion due to negative experiences in childhood. Some had a specific religion forced on them; for others, the tenets of their given religion are not reconcilable with political or ethical beliefs they have adopted as an adult. But spirituality can be found outside organized religion. A 2005 *Newsweek*/Beliefnet poll found that more Americans identify themselves as spiritual (79 percent) than religious (64 percent). If organized religion is not for you, you are not alone. Feel confident developing your own understanding of faith, spirituality, and God's presence in our lives.

Principle #150

Understand that spirituality is not in conflict with other beliefs you hold.

It is often assumed that religion and science must be at odds with one another. But one of the greatest scientists of all time, Albert Einstein, also shed light on the relationship between religion and science. Einstein believed that conflicts between science and religion were based on misunderstandings, and argued, "Science without religion is lame, religion without science is blind: a legitimate conflict between science and religion cannot exist." Keep Einstein's words in mind the next time you feel forced to choose between your faith and another belief you hold.

Principle #151

Realize that spirituality and faith are not magic tricks.

An old saying goes, "Faith can move mountains, but don't be surprised if God hands you a shovel." Indeed, do not view faith or spirituality as a magic ticket that will get you everything in life you desire. Believing in a higher power is not about wishing for a new car or petitioning for an amazing husband. It is about becoming the type of person who is worthy of such gifts. If you are to reap the benefits of spirituality, which include a more meaningful, happy, and longer life, you will have to work hard for them — but have faith you will be rewarded.

Avoiding Risky Behaviors

There are some kinds of risks that, if taken, will enhance your life beyond your wildest imagination. Investing what you can afford in the stock market, quitting the job you hate, and picking up and moving across the country for a better life all fall under the category of risks you should not be afraid to take if they fit within your goals and dreams. But there are certain risks that are not worth taking under any circumstances. These are risks that threaten to make you sick, injured, shorten your life, or hurt those around you.

In avoiding risky behaviors, you will need to become skilled at learning the difference between high risks and calculated risks. Heart-pounding activities such as skydiving, rock climbing, or SCUBA diving are calculated risks. While they pose a risk in some circumstances and can even result in death, their risk is reduced through advanced skill-building and training. Likewise, with proper knowledge, investing in the stock market or real estate is considered a calculated risk because the chances of failure can be reduced to a manageable amount.

High-risk behaviors, on the other hand, are risks in which you are more likely to lose everything and gain nothing while putting yourself and those around you in danger in the process. For example, drinking and driving is unacceptable high-risk behavior, as is gambling excessively, being careless with firearms, and being reckless with your diet.

Author Jeanette Winterson once wrote, "What you risk reveals what you value." With that in mind, when you take needless risks you show how little you value your health and happiness. Indulging in high-risk activities and behaviors is a surefire way to undo every single other effort you have made to increase your day-to-day happiness and lengthen your life. In fact, if you are to read no other chapter in this book, make sure to read this one. Use the following simple principles to avoid behaviors that will surely lead to a life of sickness, misery, and premature death.

Principle #152

Never have sex without protection.

Businessman Bob Rubin once famously joked, "Condoms aren't completely safe. A friend of mine was wearing one and got hit by a bus." It is true that condoms are not foolproof, but wearing them properly during sexual activity prevents pregnancy 98 percent of the time and diseases such as HIV and AIDS 99 percent of the time. Use condoms every time you have sex to radically reduce your risk of pregnancy, disease, and cancers that result from STDs.

PRINCIPLE #153

Know your partner's sexual history.

One in 5 Americans carries a sexually transmitted disease. Therefore, before you get in bed with someone, learn their sexual history. This is an uncomfortable topic but one that must be broached for both people's safety. You will want to ask any prospective partner the following: How many people have you slept with? Have you ever failed to use protection? Have you been tested for HIV/AIDS and when? This conversation will yield valuable information that will help you decide if it is safe for you to get in bed. To build trust, provide your partner with your own sexual history.

Principle #154

Realize you are never too old to acquire an STD.

Though teenagers and young adults are at highest risk for acquiring an STD, a person can do so at any age — all that is required is having unprotected sex with an infected person. Interestingly, as the Baby Boomer generation retires to active-adult communities, health workers have seen a dramatic increase in STDs in those populations. This is because people 55-plus were not taught sexual education as were younger Americans and fail to protect themselves with their new sexual partners. Whether you are 20, 40, 60, or 80, realize you can catch an STD if you do not practice safe sex.

Principle #155

Avoid unexpectedly expecting.

— ❄ —

Comedian Bill Maher once joked, "Kids. They're not easy. But there has to be some penalty for sex." Raising a child is difficult and when attempted under the wrong circumstances can be disastrous. Babies put a strain on even the best relationships. Furthermore, they are expensive — according to a 2004 report, it costs about $167,000 to raise a child from birth to age 18 and even more if you help pay for college. This figure does not take into account lost salary if one parent has to quit working to take care of the child. Protect your finances, relationship, and future prospects by bearing children only when you are ready and able.

PRINCIPLE #156

Never share needles.

Most people will never share intravenous needles because they are not drug addicts. But hepatitis, HIV and AIDS, and other diseases that are transmitted via intravenous needle-sharing can be contracted through more common activities as well, such as body piercing, tattooing, and even donating blood. As a rule, if a needle or sharp instrument has been in someone else's skin, don't use it. When receiving a service such as a tattoo, always check that the equipment has been sterilized and fresh needles are used.

Principle #157

Use alcohol responsibly.

Americans have a confusing relationship with alcohol. Alcohol is a potent, addictive substance that has physical, emotional, and even hallucinogenic effects, yet it is legal, readily available, and socially encouraged. When used responsibly, drinking alcohol can be a relaxing, enjoyable experience. But when abused, it can have severe consequences, including blackouts and depression. In fact, according to the Substance Abuse and Mental Health Services Administration, 37 percent of people who commit suicide have alcohol in their bloodstream. Work throughout your life to develop a safe and responsible relationship with alcohol — the risks of not doing so are too high.

Principle #158

Avoid keeping guns in the house.

— ❋ —

According to a 2005 Gallup poll, 4 in 10 Americans keep a gun in their home. Furthermore, 34 percent of children live in homes with firearms — that is more than 22 million kids. When children get their hands on guns, accidental deaths, suicides, school shootings, and other tragedies occur. If you own a gun, make sure it will not be discovered by a child or burglar. Keep your gun outside of the home. If you must keep it at home, store it unloaded in a safe, separate from the ammunition. Supplying the weapon for a criminal or accidental shooting is a risk you must not take.

Principle #159

Never drive drunk.

According to the U.S. Department of Transportation, there is an alcohol-related traffic fatality every 31 minutes and an alcohol-related traffic injury every 2 minutes. Alcohol is involved in 40 percent of fatal car accidents, and about 1.5 million drivers are arrested each year for driving under the influence of alcohol. Driving drunk can only hurt you and those in your community. Though it may seem time-consuming or expensive to call a cab, always err on the side of caution. Drunk driving has strict penalties, the harshest of which is the loss of life and freedom.

Principle #160

Consider junk food a health risk not worth taking.

It may seem strange to consider eating junk food a high-risk activity. Yet the consumption of junk food is a main cause of obesity, which was recently declared an epidemic by the National Institutes of Health. Junk food is laden with salt, calories, and fat. In fact, the average fast-food meal can contain 2,000 calories, a person's recommended intake for a whole day! The average American eats 159 fast-food meals a year, which packs on the pounds. Becoming obese increases the risk of diabetes, cardiovascular disease, heart attack, stroke, and cancer. Reduce your risk by avoiding junk food, starting today.

Looking, Feeling, and Thinking Young

The Irish playwright Oscar Wilde once wrote, "To get back my youth I would do anything in the world, except take exercise, get up early, or be respectable." Wilde knew a thing or two about the desire for eternal youth. In 1891, he wrote the classic novel *The Picture of Dorian Gray*, which was about the lengths a man will go in order to prevent aging. Wilde tapped into an enduring truth about a person's age: The extent to which you feel, think, and look old is a direct result of the way you care for your mind and body in younger years.

Some ways to stave off looking, thinking, and feeling old involve practicing basic self-care. This includes brushing and flossing regularly to maintain a youthful, white smile; practicing good posture; eating well; and exercising regularly. Each of these activities preserves the body, retaining as youthful an appearance as possible.

But perhaps the most important place to preserve the seeds of looking, thinking, and feeling young is in the mind. Keeping your mind young involves never giving up on dreams; being open to new ideas and experiences; being optimistic; and engaging in activities you loved as a younger person. As writer Edward Bulwer-Lytton once said, "It is not by the gray of the hair that one knows the age of the heart." Indeed, you can be any age if you feel, think, and look young.

Looking, thinking, and feeling young has benefits far beyond the vanity of wanting to stay slim or wrinkle-free. Studies have shown again and again that a person's mindset and activities are directly linked to how long they live. A recent study by the Mayo Clinic, for example, found that, on average, optimists live 20 percent longer than pessimists. Another study conducted by researchers at Stanford University found that the more involved people are in hobbies and activities that interest them, the longer they will live. Said Dr. Walter Bortz, professor of medicine at Stanford and leader of the study, "People who stay involved have a tendency to live longer, as they have more reasons to get out of bed in the morning."

PRINCIPLE #161

Turn back the clock with exercise.

※

There are many great reasons to make exercise a regular part of your routine, and looking and feeling younger is now among them. Researchers at the University of Texas Southwestern Medical Center studied the bodies of 50-year-old men and found that they were able to regain the aerobic capacity they had in their 20s simply by exercising several times a week for 6 months. Indeed, exercising regularly improves flexibility and muscle function. Avoid exercise-related injuries by sticking with non-impact exercises such as walking and swimming.

Principle #162

Keep up to speed with technology.

In the 21st century, it seems like there is a new technological advance every day! While it often can be overwhelming, you must keep up to date with new technologies in order to think and feel young. Take a computer course — most adult education departments offer classes on email, the Internet, and other computer functions. Get an iPod and load it with music. Experiment with websites by browsing them to get a feel for how they work. The most important thing is to be interested in our changing world — this is a surefire way not to get left behind by it.

Principle #163

Use SPF to SOW (Stave Off Wrinkles).

---※---

Using sunscreen every day is the best way to prevent wrinkles. In fact, a 2006 Consumer Reports study found that sunscreen is not only cheaper than fancy, name-brand lotions and moisturizers but more effective at preventing wrinkles. Says dermatologist Susan Weinkle, "You can use expensive wrinkle creams until the cows come home. But they aren't going to do much good if you don't protect your face from sun damage." Therefore, incorporate sunscreen into your daily skin care routine. Apply an oil-free facial sunscreen or buy a moisturizer with sunscreen included. Men should look for skin care lines made expressly for them to prevent age-telling lines.

Principle #164

Never limit yourself based on your age.

— ✳ —

Don't use your age as an excuse for not doing things! It is never too late to get an advanced degree, travel to an exotic land, or learn a new craft. The only thing preventing you from such adventure is your preconceived notion that these activities are for young people. In fact, retirees account for an increasing percentage of the nation's students and adventure-travel companies host 55-plus trips to places as varied as China and Brazil. Pigeonholing yourself into a particular age bracket is a surefire way to be confined to it. As it is often said, "Middle age is when we can do just as much as ever — but would rather not."

Principle #165

Resurrect hobbies you loved when you were young.

Poet Oliver Wendell Holmes once quipped, "Men do not quit playing because they grow old; they grow old because they quit playing." To throw off the cobwebs of an older mindset, don't give up on the hobbies you loved in your younger years. If you played an instrument, start practicing; if you loved to paint, dig out your brushes and canvas. Engaging in the activities you loved as a younger person is an excellent way to jump-start your creativity and feel better about yourself.

Principle #166

Stay hydrated.

To look younger than your years, it is essential to stay hydrated. In fact, once a person turns 57, their body literally starts to dry up! Studies have shown that the bodies of those in their late-50s are composed of just 54 percent water versus younger bodies that are composed of 61 percent water or more. As we age, our sweat glands shrivel, causing us to sweat less. This puts us at risk for overheating and heatstroke. Taking in more water can prevent against these conditions. Finally, staying hydrated prevents skin wrinkles, which truly show your age.

Principle #167

Realize you are never too old to follow through on your dreams.

The great Russian writer Anton Chekhov suffered from tuberculosis. At 37, the disease became debilitating and doctors ordered him to rest, fearing he had not much longer to live. With this news, Chekhov did not lie down and wait for death. Instead, he pursued his dream of building a summer home in the region of Yalta. He bought a plot, built a home, and beautified the land with flowers and fruit trees. Chekhov died just 5 years later, but his inspiring story reminds us to make the most of our time on earth and follow our dreams, no matter how much time remains.

Principle #168

Feel young by counting your experience, not your years.

American writer Madeleine L'Engle once said, "The great thing about getting older is that you don't lose all the other ages you've been." Indeed, recognize that with each year you add wisdom, laughter, and experience to the sum of who you are. Think of yourself not as 50, but as 20 with 30 years of experience! Your young mindset, coupled with your maturity, will make you feel great about yourself and make others drawn to you.

Principle #169

Be silly!

Doug Larson once said, "The aging process has you firmly in its grasp if you never get the urge to throw a snowball." A lifelong racecar driver, Larson knew a thing or two about the importance of having fun. Take Larson's advice and have fun no matter what your age! Throw a snowball, make a funny face, do a dance, or wear a funny costume — embrace being silly as the most fun way to look, feel, and think young.

Principle #170

Keep an open mind.

Our years of hard-won experience are wonderful when they help us learn from our mistakes and avoid obvious pitfalls. But when our experience prevents us from thinking openly about opportunities or ideas, we become trapped rather than informed by it. Avoid the curmudgeonly, know-it-all, old personality we all hated as youths. Instead, keep an open mind no matter what your age. Remind yourself that society changes very quickly, and some of your experiences may no longer apply to the current context. Be prepared to learn something new every day. As Henry Ford once said, "Anyone who stops learning is old, whether at 20 or 80."

PRINCIPLE #171

Develop a young philosophy of life.

———————————— ✳ ————————————

It doesn't matter how old you are if your philosophy of life is young. This means seeing the world through the most youthful lens of all: optimism. Indeed, young people are young because they still believe everything is possible and that all problems can be solved. While you needn't deny the certain truths you have learned in life, you will benefit by incorporating a certain degree of optimism into your outlook. As General Douglas MacArthur once put it, "You are as young as your faith, as old as your doubt; as young as your self-confidence, as old as your fear; as young as your hope, as old as your despair."

Principle #172

Be proud of your age.

While working on looking, thinking, and feeling young, never attempt to deny your age. Trying to deny the fact that you have been around the block will only cause others to view you as older than you are. Grow old gracefully by approaching the issue of age from Mark Twain's perspective when he wrote: "Age is an issue of mind over matter. If you don't mind, it doesn't matter." Above all, never regret growing older — it is, after all, a privilege not everyone enjoys.

Nurturing Friendships

In 2005, a groundbreaking research study published in the Journal of Epidemiology and Community Health found that having a network of good friends, rather than family, can extend a person's life span. After studying thousands of people for more than a decade, researchers found that close contact with children and relatives has little impact on how long a person lives. However, a close network of good friends and confidants significantly improved a person's chances of surviving longer.

One reason for the life-giving benefits of friendship is that friends often affect each others' behavior in positive ways, especially as they get older. Friends, more often than relatives, are likely to be the source of a person's social contact and thus have more of a chance to influence their behavior. If a person's friends eat healthy, refrain from smoking, and drink occasionally, so too will a person who spends time with them.

Likewise, friends often bond over shared physical activities, such as walking or playing a game of tennis or golf, which keep a person healthy and living longer.

But friends also provide something that family members often do not: a supportive, nonjudgmental, accepting environment that helps a person cope with frustration, difficulty, sadness, and loss. Friends nurture talents and interests in each other that family sometimes fails to appreciate; they also tend to "get" each other in a way that family often do not. These emotional connections are clearly important for feeling better and living longer. In fact, friendship is one of the explanations for why women live longer than men. Studies have shown that women are far more likely than men to make friends, keep friendships longer, and to form friendships over more diverse activities. In 2004, life expectancy for American women was 5.2 years longer than men — many scientists suspect their adeptness at making and retaining friends explains why.

But no matter your gender, your ability to make, nurture, and keep friendships will directly affect how good you feel on a daily basis and even how long you live. With this as your goal, use the following principles to surround yourself with excellent friends.

PRINCIPLE #173

Seek meaningful interactions with friends.

Our fast-paced society makes it hard to find time for meaningful interactions with people. It is easy to dash off a quick email, leave a voicemail, or text a message and then feel like you have made the effort to connect. These superficial communications are no substitute for true interaction. In order to develop real friendships, you must put time and energy into nurturing them. So meet your friend for coffee, a drink, or a round of golf. Send him or her a handwritten birthday card in the mail. Going these extra lengths will endear you to the people you care about most.

Principle #174

Do favors for your friends.

— ❊ —

Friends are wonderful gifts, and they should be rewarded now and then without having to ask. If you know a friend is moving, offer to help box up his belongings. Consider house-sitting while your pal goes on a much-needed vacation. Or, make dinner for your friend and take it to her when she gets home from a rough day at work. You will both benefit from these small kindnesses. Act in the spirit of French philosopher Albert Camus' words: "Friendship isn't a big thing — it's a million little things."

Principle #175

Be an honest friend.

The mark of a true friend is someone who is willing to say or hear something unpleasant. For example, if you listen to your chronically late friend complain about her boss's bad mood, point out that she could make the situation better by showing up to work and meetings on time. Being unquestioningly supportive might make you an easy confidant, but it does not make you a true friend. To do your friends a service you must be willing to point out the stuff they might prefer to ignore. As an old Sicilian proverb goes, "Only your real friends will tell you when your face is dirty."

Principle #176

Give your friendships room to grow.

Most friendships are born from sharing a common experience or hobby. Some friends meet at work, others bond over a shared class, hobby, or life situation. While initial friendships will be tied to the circumstance that brought them together, it is important to stay close with your friends once you no longer share that common denominator. Work to embrace your friend's new situation; be in step with a friend even if you are no longer on the same page of life. As author Elisabeth Foley has written, "The most beautiful discovery true friends make is that they can grow separately without growing apart."

Principle #177

Avoid keeping score.

Keeping score in a friendship is never productive. Do favors and tasks out of love and responsibility, not to have ammunition for future debates. Likewise, never do things for a friend solely so they will someday have to repay you. As Hubert Humphrey once said, "If you keep score on the good things and the bad things, you'll find out that you're a very miserable person. God gave man the ability to forget, which is one of the greatest attributes you have. Because if you remember everything that's happened to you, you generally remember that which is the most unfortunate." To stay happy in your friendships, refrain from keeping score.

Principle #178

Honor the plans you make with your friends.

If you make plans with your friends, keep them. Skipping out on a commitment tells your friends they are not important to you. If every year your friend hosts a July Fourth barbecue, put it on your calendar and make sure you attend. Honoring smaller commitments are just as important. Birthday dinners, casual lunches, sport games, and other outings are all chances to show your friends how much you value their presence in your life.

Principle #179

Show your friends you are sorry.

---- ❋ ----

Everyone makes mistakes in life, but not everyone knows how to take responsibility when they mess up. Accepting responsibility for your words and actions (even when unintentional) is an important part of having successful friendships. Humanitarian Werner Erhard wrote, "Being responsible starts with the willingness to deal with a situation from the view of life that you are the generator of what you do, what you have and what you are." So when you misspeak, correct yourself. When you err, recognize it and apologize. Your friends will appreciate your willingness to apologize when you are at fault.

Principle #180

Be an available friend.

Maintaining friendships can sometimes take a lot of work! You must be willing to invest your time in phone calls, parties, games, outings, and one-on-one time. To make good friends and enjoy their support, you must be available for them when they need you. Realize that it takes a lot of work to have close friends, and be willing to make time, at any hour, to be a good friend. As the poet Robert Brault once quipped, "I value the friend who for me finds time on his calendar, but I cherish the friend who for me does not consult his calendar."

Principle #181

Take opportunities to make new friends.

Author Rod McKuen once remarked, "Strangers are just friends waiting to happen." Indeed, there is no better time to make a new friend than today! If you are lonely for new friends, strike up conversation with someone you meet at a party. Pursue people you know through professional or social networks. Attend an event in your community, such as a lecture or reading that will bring you in contact with people who share your interests. Making friends takes putting yourself out there — once you do, you are sure to be surrounded by many interesting people.

PRINCIPLE #182

Realize that good friends stick around for the hard stuff.

It's easy to be someone's friend when it means going to parties and laughing the time away. But the mark of a true friend is one who makes him or herself available to someone during a dark or challenging time. Many people fear this time of friendship because they don't know how to be comforting or fear saying the wrong thing. If this applies to you, think of what author Barbara Kingsolver has written: "The friend who holds your hand and says the wrong thing is made of dearer stuff than the one who stays away."

Principle #183

Learn to accept apologies from friends.

— ❊ —

Accepting an apology is a tricky art that must be mastered to have successful friendships. First, you must let the other person know that their actions or words have hurt you. Hopefully, your friend will apologize. If you want to continue the relationship, you will have to accept the apology. The difficult part is letting the apology saturate your relationship. This means you absorb it completely and let the incident go. Accept the inevitability that, at times, friends will hurt each others' feelings. You will feel better if you are able to express yourself, accept an apology, and move on.

Principle #184

Strive for jealousy-free friendships.

Jealousy is the great friendship destroyer. There may be reasons to envy your friends, but succumbing to jealousy will create distance in your relationships. Coveting your friend's big house or attentive partner will shrink your capacity to love and support him. Jealously guarding your friend and being unwilling to share her with others is likely to foster resentment and secrecy. Support the friends you have wholeheartedly so that they will want to support you when good fortune comes your way.

Principle #185

Realize that some friendships have expiration dates.

Sadly, not all the friends you make will be friends for life. While you should try to nurture your friendships, it is also important to recognize when you simply don't have enough in common with someone anymore. At that point, the relationship may be time-consuming, frustrating, or even painful for you. If so, you must accept that some friendships have expiration dates — in other words, the relationship served you well for a certain phase of your life but no longer contributes in a meaningful or positive way. In such a case, let the friendship go and save your energy for your more enduring relationships.

Principle #186

Above all, make friends with yourself.

---※---

The relationship you have with yourself is the foundation for the friendships you make with others. If you are miserable and seek to find joy only in others, you will always be looking for happiness in the wrong place. Furthermore, if you dislike yourself, potential friends will have no reason to like you. Indeed, the love and respect you have for yourself is directly proportional to the love and respect your friends are able to feel for you. As actress Lucille Ball once said, "Love yourself first and everything else falls into line."

Coping with Sadness

No book on how to feel better and live a longer life would be complete without addressing the presence of sadness in our lives. Coping with sadness is a challenge many of us face daily to varying degrees.

Learning how to cope with separation, death, and other serious problems that cause sadness is necessary for your survival. In fact, as of 2007, there have been nearly a dozen studies from reputable institutions such as Yale University that show that people who avoid sadness live longer and healthier lives. One study found that they are less likely to suffer heart attacks, strokes, and experience pain from conditions like arthritis. In another study, researchers from Carnegie Mellon University found that happy people come down with fewer colds and flus than those who are consumed with negative emotions such as anger, sadness, or stress. Becoming a happier person is so important that in 2006, Harvard University developed an entire course on how to become happy. More than 850 students enrolled, making it the university's most popular class.

There are many ways to manage your sadness. First, though, you must assess whether you are sad or depressed. If you are depressed, see a doctor or therapist, because you may need a professional to help guide you. If you are experiencing a proportionate level of sadness to a particular event, you will be able to be feel better again if you take care not to let your sadness spiral out of control. The Lebanese-American poet Kahlil Gibran once wrote, "Sadness is but a wall between two gardens." In this spirit, use the following principles to learn how to cope with sadness and return to your garden of happiness. Doing so will ensure you live a long, happy, and healthy life.

PRINCIPLE #187

Learn how to cry.

Humans are the only animals that shed tears as a result of emotions. But there are many of us who never allow ourselves to cry. Some are afraid of being embarrassed while others bottle up their sadness in an attempt to feel it less. Avoiding the process of crying is unhealthy, says Dr. Barry M. Bernfeld, director of the Primal Institute. Bernfeld has found that crying relieves stress and even removes waste products and toxic substances from the body. "Crying is natural, healthy and curative," says Bernfeld. "We seem finally to recognize that crying is good for people." So allow yourself to have a good, cathartic cry now and then.

Principle #188

Mourn when your loss is fresh.

— ❊ —

When a loved one dies, many of us go into survival mode. Things need to be done, so we do them. It feels like as long as you keep moving and doing, you will be OK. This state of autopilot might carry you through the initial shock but can lead to a crushing collapse as time goes on. So when faced with loss, allow yourself time to grieve in the immediate aftermath of the event. Do what needs to be done, but also remain in touch with your feelings; process your loss by moving forward through each stage of grief and in time you will recover.

Principle #189

Avoid letting sadness define you.

If we allow sadness to permeate every aspect of our lives, it begins to affect the people around us. Allowing sadness to define who we are is dangerous, as it promises to rob us of many joys and even cuts our lives short. Work through your sadness instead of letting it spill over into every area of your life. As a Chinese proverb says, "You cannot prevent the birds of sadness from passing over your head, but you can prevent their making a nest in your hair." Be mindful of your sadness and prevent it from becoming a permanent feature of your life.

Principle #190

Develop coping skills for everyday problems.

Learn to deal with life's little curveballs in order to stand tall when the big pitches are thrown. It makes sense that people who have trouble coping with the setbacks of daily life will have a more difficult time recovering from serious trauma and loss. Start working on your coping skills today so you are better prepared in case you are faced with a major tragedy. Learning how to deal with small setbacks will help you avoid coming completely unglued when something big happens, because you will have a larger selection of coping tools from which to choose.

Principle #191

Realize there is no timetable for grieving.

Everyone mourns on their own schedule. For some people the passage of time makes their loss easier. Others find that anniversaries, birthdays, and other milestones are painful reminders that can make their loss feel as if it has just occurred. However long it takes you to find a comfortable pace for mourning your loss is the correct amount of time. Avoid berating yourself for taking too long to get over your tragedy. This will only add guilt on top of pain and increase your stress level. Be gentle with yourself and allow your grieving process to unfold naturally.

Principle #192

Reminisce about a loved one.

Gather with friends and family and tell stories about the person whom you've lost. This practice will both honor the person who died and help express your feelings in a healthy way. It is not productive to deny the deceased person's existence. Eventually, missing him or her will creep up on you when you least expect it, unhealthily interrupting your daily routine. As the Roman poet Ovid once wrote, "Suppressed grief suffocates, it rages within the breast, and is forced to multiply its strength." So talk about those you miss — they would have wanted it that way.

Principle #193

Understand that grief is an individual experience.

There is no perfect way to grieve, though there are general phases people go through. In 1969, Elisabeth Kübler-Ross established the 5 stages of grief: denial, anger, bargaining, depression, and acceptance. However, even Kübler-Ross said these were basic guidelines and not strict rules for grieving. In 2004, she said, "They were never meant to help tuck messy emotions into neat packages. … There is not a typical response to loss, as there is no typical loss. Our grief is as individual as our lives." Don't worry if your grieving process doesn't match anyone else's — grief is as varied as humans are.

PRINCIPLE #194

Use humor to lighten the darkest mood.

———————————— ✳ ————————————

American humorist Irvin S. Cobb once wrote, "Humor is merely tragedy standing on its head with its pants torn." Without downplaying your sadness, find relief by exploring the humorous side of things. If you are down because you have recently been fired, think of funny stories from your work instead of focusing on your lost job. If your sadness stems from the loss of a loved one, think of what would make him laugh if he were with you. Laughing in the midst of darkness is not disrespectful to your sadness but rather shines a light for a brief and healing moment.

PRINCIPLE #195

Let friends and family care for you when you are down.

---- ✳ ----

Everyone needs help sometimes. When you are feeling sad and find you have trouble coping, let your friends and family help you. They can do simple things, such as bring you dinner or do a load of laundry. A family member or close friend can also help you remember who you were before the tragic event occurred. Mourning alone is taxing and can even become dangerous if you lose touch with the outside world. In your darkest times, be sure to allow those who love you to help out.

Principle #196

Find a creative outlet
to express your feelings.

When you are down, the last thing you feel like doing is being creative. But as the artist Corita Kent said, "Flowers grow from dark moments." When you are sad, try writing a poem or story about the event that has you down. If you are a visual person, draw or paint, using colors that capture your mood. If you are more crafty, start a project that can take your mind off your problems. Expressing your feelings in a new and creative way will help you feel better more quickly.

Principle #197

Start new traditions to honor a person you've lost.

Keep alive the memory of those who have passed by integrating them into your holidays and traditions. For example, make one of your grandmother's favorite dishes a new staple at the Thanksgiving table. Raise a glass and toast to your father on his birthday and tell his favorite story from when you were growing up. What was your grandmother's favorite charity? Make a donation in her name every year. There are many ways to invoke lost loved ones when you find yourself missing them.

Principle #198

Don't be afraid to feel sad.

Author Jim Rohn writes, "The walls we build around us to keep sadness out also keeps out the joy." Indeed, sadness is one of the many human emotions that we need to feel in order to keep a healthy emotional balance. It is impossible to escape sadness — but you can minimize its effect on your life by acknowledging you feel sad at certain times. Bottling up sadness is not healthy for anyone — so don't be afraid to feel sad from time to time.

Principle #199

Know the difference between sadness and depression.

---   ✳   ---

Sadness is a normal response to a loss or tragedy. Sad feelings will usually pass after a certain amount of time, but left unchecked, sadness can turn into depression. Depression often requires treatment such as therapy and sometimes medication. If you feel unable to cope with your daily activities, avoid friends and family, or are unable to care for yourself, seek help. According to the American Psychiatric Association, "Depression is never normal and always produces needless suffering. With proper diagnosis and treatment, the vast majority of people with depression will overcome it." Treating depression is important for feeling better again.

Principle #200

Remember that sadness is part of the human experience.

Sociologist Emile Durkheim wrote, "Man could not live if he were entirely impervious to sadness." It is true that sadness is an important part of the natural life cycle. It often takes something tragic to make us realize all that we have to be thankful for. Sadness can also be an opportunity to reach out to those around us, which ultimately enriches our lives. Don't panic if you are feeing down — take a deep breath and remember that you are only human. You will feel better again, and this, too, shall pass.

ADDITIONAL INFORMATION AND IDEAS

The following pages contain a few exercises that will help you feel better and live longer. Practicing these exercises will help you develop a lifestyle that allows you to make the most out of life!

These exercises will help you overcome habits that are preventing you from feeling your best. Make a habit of performing them whenever you are feeling particularly lethargic or unhealthy. They will also help you get back on track with your physical, mental, dietary, and emotional goals.

Practice these exercises to become familiar with healthy foods, feel stress-free, and achieve mental health and confidence. Each of these skills must be mastered if you are to feel your best and live a long life.

The following should be practiced daily to feel better and live longer:

Ten Exercises — Ten Minutes Each
These exercises can maximize flexibility, strength, and muscle tone. Each can be done in less than 10 minutes.

Foods To Make You Feel Better and Live Longer
Eat at least 1 serving of 5 to 8 of these foods every day to reduce the risk of cancer, heart disease, diabetes, stroke, and hypertension.

Ideas for Relaxation
This exercise offers you quick, easy, and unique ideas for achieving a relaxed state.

Replacements for Soda
Chemicals in soda have been linked to many diseases. Instead of soda, reach for one of the following drinks.

Positive Affirmations
Repeat the affirmations in this exercise to start feeling better about yourself immediately.

Ten Exercises — Ten Minutes Each

Choose several of the following exercises every day to maximize flexibility, strength, and muscle tone. Each can be done in less than 10 minutes – some can even be done while watching television! You have no excuse for not incorporating them into your daily routine

1) Go for a walk
2) Learn 5 yoga poses and practice them
3) Jump up and down 20 to 30 times
4) Do 3 sets of 40 sit-ups
5) Do 3 sets of 40 push-ups
6) Run up and down a flight of stairs
7) Stretch each quadrant of your body
8) Ride a bicycle
9) Squat repeatedly
10) Dance around the house while singing

Foods to Make You Feel Better and Live Longer

Each of the following foods contains vitamins and minerals that have been proven to prevent or reduce cancer, heart disease, diabetes, stroke, and hypertension. Eat at least 1 serving of 5 to 8 of them every day. In pencil, put a checkmark next to each food when you have eaten it. Try to mark off each food at least once a week. After the week is up, erase your marks and start again (* denotes a Super Food, or food that is particularly excellent for either losing weight, fighting disease, or extending life span).

Apples

Artichokes

Asparagus

Avocados

Bananas

Bell peppers

Beans/legumes*

Blackberries

Blueberries*

Broccoli*

Brown rice

Buckwheat

Cantaloupe

Cauliflower

Chicken

Cranberries

Carrots

Chili peppers

Cheese

Eggplant

Eggs

Garlic

Ginger

Grapefruit

Lean meat

Oats*

Olive oil

Oranges*

Milk

Nuts*

Peaches

Pineapples

Peas

Pumpkin*

Quinoa

Salmon*

Soy*

Spinach*

Strawberries

Tea*

Tempeh

Tofu

Tomatoes*

Tuna

Turkey*

Whole wheat products

Yogurt*

Water

IDEAS FOR RELAXATION

1. Inhale and exhale deeply and very slowly 10 times.
2. Stretch your back and legs by reaching to your toes with your fingers without bending your knees. Go as far down as you can.
3. Lie flat on your back, close your eyes, and stretch your arms and toes out away from each other.
4. Starting from your shoulders, progressively relax each muscle group by stretching and releasing tension, ending with your toes.
5. Take a warm bath.
6. Get a massage.
7. Light candles.
8. Have a warm cup of herbal tea.
9. Massage your own scalp.
10. Close your eyes for 10 minutes during the day and think positive thoughts.
11. Exercise for at least 30 minutes each day.

12. Practice yoga.
13. Practice Tai Chi.
14. Go for a walk in the sunshine.
15. Use aromatherapy.
16. Listen to soothing music.
17. Meditate.
18. Get enough sleep.

REPLACEMENTS FOR SODA

Chemicals in soda have been linked to diseases such as cancer, diabetes, obesity, hypertension, and osteoporosis. If you drink soda, begin working immediately to wean yourself off it. Instead of reaching for soda, try any one of the following drinks (* indicates caffeinated beverage).

Herbal tea
Black or green tea*
Yerba matte tea*
Ice water
Water flavored with fruit slices
Natural fruit juice
Organic coffee
Iced tea*
Hot cocoa
Sparkling water
Lemonade

Positive Affirmations

Replacing negative thoughts with positive ones is one of the best ways to feel better about ourselves. Furthermore, studies have shown that thinking positively increases life span by up to 19 percent! So tell yourself something from this list several times a day. Look in a mirror while you say the affirmation. Focus on the words and how it feels to say positive statements about yourself. When you feel the urge to say, "This is stupid," force yourself to replace that thought with one of the affirmations below.

- I am smart.
- I am capable.
- I am learning.
- I am trying my best.
- I am a good person.
- I am fun.
- I like myself.
- I love myself.
- I forgive myself.

- I am good at what I do.
- I like what I do.
- I am happy.
- I am loving.
- I am kind.
- I am grateful.
- I accept my flaws.
- I have many strengths.
- I deserve to be happy.
- I am becoming more healthy every day.
- I am a work in progress.
- I am important.
- I like my body.
- My body is perfectly imperfect.
- I respect myself.
- I deserve respect from others.
- I am proud of myself.
- Everything is going to work out.
- The steps I take today will improve my tomorrow.
- I will succeed.

CONCLUSION

Congratulations! After reading this book you should feel good about your prospects for living a longer, happier, and healthier life. There are an infinite number of ways to extend your life span, but the fastest manner to achieve this is by starting today to change your lifestyle in order to maximize your longevity and minimize your pain. If you smoke, stop now; if you eat unhealthily, eat better; if you avoid exercise, find a form of it you enjoy. These are the basic pillars of feeling better and living longer, and this book provides you with more than 200 other ideas, tips, tricks, and pieces of advice for extending your life.

Simple Principles™ to Feel Better and Live Longer gives you the tools to deal with an increasingly toxic world that makes it challenging to live a healthy life. It also gives you hundreds of reasons why you should want to feel better and live longer. Remember that sacrificing your mental and physical health today will hurt you tomorrow. Learn to navigate the many hazards and pitfalls the world throws at you in order to feel your best and live a longer life.

As you apply the wisdom in this book to feel better and live longer, it is important to remember every day that you are changing your whole life for the better. Some of these benefits will be seen immediately. For example, increasing your intake of water will make your body function better in under a week. Likewise, learning deep breathing exercises and yoga postures can envelope you in relaxation and calm in under 5 minutes! Other changes will take longer to benefit from, but they are just as important to pursue. For example, having close friends extends your life by years, but it can also take years to cultivate friendships. Or, eating antioxidants over time can reduce your risk of cancer, but you may not win that battle for decades to come. No matter which aspect of feeling better and living longer you work on, know that your hard work will pay off, and you will be glad you did it!

Above all, practice what you have learned in this book often. Keep it handy and refer to it when you need a reminder or a pick-me-up. A healthier, happier, longer life is completely within your grasp if you adopt the new habits and ways of thinking presented in this book. Remember, you deserve to feel better and live longer!

Great Titles in the
SIMPLE PRINCIPLES™ SERIES

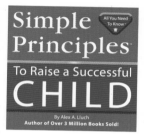

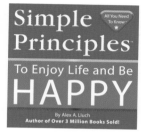

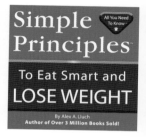

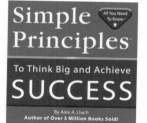

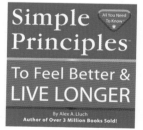

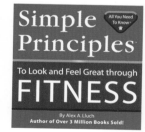

LOG ON TO **WSPublishingGroup.com** TO CHECK FOR
RELEASE DATES ON THESE AND FUTURE TITLES.

More Great Titles in the
SIMPLE PRINCIPLES™ SERIES

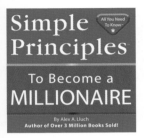

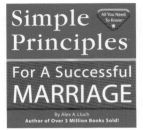

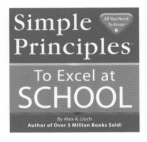

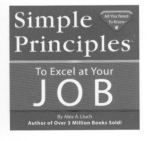

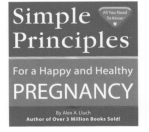

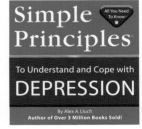

LOG ON TO **WSPublishingGroup.com** TO CHECK FOR
RELEASE DATES ON THESE AND FUTURE TITLES.

Other Best-Selling Books by Alex A. Lluch

HOME & FINANCE

- The Very Best Home Improvement Guide & Document Organizer
- The Very Best Home Buying Guide & Document Organizer
- The Very Best Home Selling Guide & Document Organizer
- The Very Best Budget & Finance Guide with Document Organizer
- The Ultimate Home Journal & Organizer
- The Ultimate Home Buying Guide & Organizer

BABY JOURNALS & PARENTING

- The Complete Baby Journal Organizer & Keepsake
- Keepsake of Love Baby Journal
- Snuggle Bears Baby Journal Keepsake & Organizer
- Humble Bumbles Baby Journal
- Simple Principles to Raise a Successful Child

CHILDREN'S BOOKS

- I Like to Learn: Alphabet, Numbers, Colors & Opposites
- Alexander, It's Time for Bed!
- Do I Look Good in Color?
- Zoo Clues Animal Alphabet
- Animal Alphabet: Slide & Seek the ABC's
- Counting Chameleon
- Big Bugs, Small Bugs

LOG ON TO **WSPublishingGroup.com** TO CHECK FOR RELEASE DATES ON THESE AND FUTURE TITLES.

More Best-Selling Books
by Alex A. Lluch

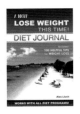

COOKING, FITNESS & DIET

- The Very Best Cooking Guide & Recipe Organizer
- Easy Cooking Guide & Recipe Organizer
- Get Fit Now! Workout Journal
- Lose Weight Now! Diet Journal & Organizer
- I Will Lose Weight This Time! Diet Journal
- The Ultimate Pocket Diet Journal

WEDDING PLANNING

- The Ultimate Wedding Planning Kit
- The Complete Wedding Planner & Organizer
- Easy Wedding Planner, Organizer & Keepsake
- Easy Wedding Planning Plus
- Easy Wedding Planning
- The Ultimate Wedding Workbook & Organizer
- The Ultimate Wedding Planner & Organizer
- Making Your Wedding Beautiful, Memorable & Unique
- Planning the Most Memorable Wedding on Any Budget
- My Wedding Journal, Organizer & Keepsake
- The Ultimate Wedding Planning Guide
- The Ultimate Guide to Wedding Music
- Wedding Party Responsibility Cards

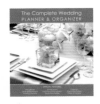

LOG ON TO **WSPublishingGroup.com** TO CHECK FOR RELEASE DATES ON THESE AND FUTURE TITLES.

About the Author and Creator of the
SIMPLE PRINCIPLES™ SERIES

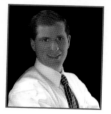

Alex A. Lluch is a seasoned entrepreneur with outstanding life achievements. He grew up very poor and lost his father at age 15. But through hard work and dedication, he has become one of the most successful authors and businessmen of our time. He is now using his life experience to write the simple principles™ series to help people improve their lives.

The following are a few of Alex's achievements:

- Author of over 3 million books sold in a wide range of categories: health, fitness, diet, home, finance, weddings, children, and babies
- President of WS Publishing Group, a successful publishing company
- President of WeddingSolutions.com, one of the world's most popular wedding planning websites
- President of UltimateGiftRegistry.com, an extensive website that allows users to register for gifts for all occasions
- President of a highly successful toy and candy company
- Has worked extensively in China, Hong Kong, Spain, Israel and Mexico
- Designed complex communication systems for Fortune 500 companies
- Black belt in Karate and Judo, winning many national tournaments
- Owns real estate in California, Colorado, Georgia and Montana
- B.S. in Electronics Engineering and an M.S. in Computer Science

Alex Lluch lives in San Diego, California with his wife of 16 years and their three wonderful children.

About the Co-Author

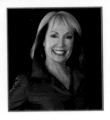 **Dr. Helen Eckmann** is a renowned expert in leadership, marketing, management and education. She has vast experience teaching in these fields as well as working with both small companies and Fortune 500 corporations. She is now sharing her insight and expertise in the 200 principles contained in this book.

The following are a few of Helen's achievements:

- Doctorate in Education and Leadership Science
- Masters in Organizational Leadership and bachelors in Management
- Consults Fortune 500 companies on leadership development
- Travels as a popular motivational speaker and mentor
- Designs and implements corporate supply chain management programs
- Serves as an Organizational Behavior Consultant to various industries
- Teaches graduate courses in business at the University of San Diego
- Has taught leadership, marketing, strategic planning, innovations and ethics to over 1,500 M.B.A. students
- Has been personnel director for several companies
- Serves on the board of directors of multiple organizations
- Founded and serves on the board of several non-profit organizations
- Provides spiritual direction to hundreds of women as a church pastor

Dr. Helen Eckmann lives with her husband in Del Mar, California. They have raised four successful children.